YOUR KID BELONGS HERE

YOUR
KID
BELONGS
HERE

**AN INSIDER'S GUIDE TO PARENTING
NEURODIVERSE CHILDREN**

Katie Rose Guest Pryal

JOHNS HOPKINS UNIVERSITY PRESS
Baltimore

Johns Hopkins University Press
2715 North Charles Street
Baltimore, Maryland 21218
www.press.jhu.edu

Library of Congress Cataloging-in-Publication Data

Names: Pryal, Katie Rose Guest, author
Title: Your kid belongs here : an insider's guide to parenting neurodiverse
    children / Katie Rose Guest Pryal.
Description: Baltimore : Johns Hopkins University Press, 2025. | Includes
    bibliographical references and index.
Identifiers: LCCN 2025003897 | ISBN 9781421453347 (hardcover) |
    ISBN 9781421453354 (paperback) | ISBN 9781421453361 (ebook)
Subjects: LCSH: Parents of autistic children | Autistic children—Family
    relationships Neurodivergent children—Family relationships | Parenting
Classification: LCC HQ773.8 .P79 2025 | DDC 649.154—dc23/eng/20250616
LC record available at https://lccn.loc.gov/2025003897

A catalog record for this book is available from the British Library.

*Special discounts are available for bulk purchases of this book. For more
information, please contact Special Sales at specialsales@jh.edu.*

EU GPSR Authorized Representative
LOGOS EUROPE, 9 rue Nicolas Poussin
17000, La Rochelle, France
E-mail: Contact@logoseurope.eu

For every neurodivergent family out there,
including mine

Contents

Preface

I never thought I'd write about my kids.

I've been a writer my entire adult life. As a poet and essayist, I've published in a wide array of literary magazines. As a clerk for a federal judge, I assisted him in drafting judicial opinions that are now public record. As a doctoral student and professor, I wrote articles for scholarly journals and books for academic audiences. Now, as a full-time writer, I've written novels, essay collections, and articles for magazines.

So many words and, until just a few years ago, not a single one was about my kids.

Why not?

Many reasons. Sometimes I write about controversial subjects, and angry readers attack me. The reader-mob on the internet attacks all writers, yes, but it attacks vulnerable writers in particular. As a neurodivergent woman, I am attacked on two fronts. Although I rarely stir up big trouble, it happens. Having my children exist online would make them targets, too, so I kept them off completely. Not only did I avoid writing about them, but I kept them off my social media: I never posted photos of their faces and never used their names. (The privacy settings on social media are unreliable at best and a joke at worst.)

As a mother-who-writes, though, not writing about my children meant that eighty percent of my life was off-limits. I write about depression—but I can't mention my near-deadly bout of postpartum depression because that would mean mentioning my children. I write about when my cat was attacked by a coyote (she lived, the glorious, spiteful thing), but I can't mention how the event affected my older child, who is, in a word, *obsessed* with cats. I write about work/life balance, but I can't write about the "life" side of things except in the vaguest of terms because for me, like for many parents, *life* means *children*.

But there was another problem that stood in the way: I'd read many social media posts, essays, op-eds, and memoirs in which parents tell deeply personal stories about their children, and the stories often made me uncomfortable. The worst of them, which seemed to dominate the public conversation, were those in which the authors revealed secrets in order to show how hard they have it as parents, using their children as foils to their own saintliness, determination, or heroism. The problem, I realized, could be summed up in one word: exploitation. So I struggled to find a middle ground between protecting my children's privacy and telling stories about my own life.

One day, everything changed. In 2017, I read an essay by Nicole Chung, a memoirist and parent of an autistic child, that shifted my perspective. In it, she detailed her fears about accessible schooling for her child because, under the (first) Trump administration, threats to disability education loomed large.[1] At one point, Chung stepped back from the thread of the essay and expressed her own concerns about writing about her child:

> I'm never sure how to write about this, or if I should even try
> at all. In our deeply ableist society, my experiences, feelings,
> and fears as a neurotypical parent are not the ones that need
> to be elevated. But it is also true that concern for our child is
> always there without me having to summon it, circling my
> mind in an unbroken loop.

Her words hit me like a brick. I came to two life-changing realizations.

The first realization was this: My kids—who are both neurodivergent, like I am—don't just take up the life side of the work/life imbalance. They permeate everything, creating the unbroken loop Chung describes. Every choice I make, they are a part of. When I sit down to write, I first make sure that they're cared for. When I quit work for the day, I seek them out. They are an atmospheric presence made up of love and, yes, anxiety for their well-being. Their presence shapes how I see the world one hundred percent of the time.

The second realization came when I read Chung's discussion of her own writing uncertainties. She approached her essay with such care, writing about her child in such a delicate ballet. Reading Chung's essay, I knew that it was possible to write about neurodiversity and parenthood without exploiting children.

In 2018, I started writing about my kids. But I never stopped struggling with the issue of exploitation. I began with a magazine column about being a neurodivergent mom of neurodivergent kids—edited, serendipitously, by Nicole Chung. In it, I told story after story about how the world doesn't make space for kids like mine—kids like yours.

But, in my very first essay, I made some mistakes. I wrote the following cringe-worthy words about my dislike of what I called the "disability parent" genre, which I described like this:

> So many essays, books, and blog posts [are] eager to overshare and, often, make money off their kids' disabilities . . . where parents talk about how great they are for parenting their children. At worst, it creates monsters: parents who feel justified emotionally or physically abusing their disabled children because their disabled children make them miserable. They

describe how awful their lives are, often on social media, and a chorus of other parents support their ableism—sometimes to the point of enabling more abuse.[2]

When I read these words now, I feel ashamed because I sound so smug, as though I believe that I am above making mistakes when I write about my kids. (I'm not.) Also, this observation had nothing at all to do with the point of the essay. Instead, I was revealing my own fears on the page. Some parents who write about their neurodivergent children do, indeed, enable more abuse, as other writers have pointed out.[3] These stories are horrific, and they deserve to be critiqued. As parents, we must understand that the responsibility we take on when we write about our neurodivergent kids is a big one.

Looking back on that first essay and the scathing critique I made of other parent-writers, I realize that I disliked the stories because it was too easy to see myself in the place of the children they feature. In the essay, I wrote, "How would I feel, I always thought, if my own parents had written about me? I believed myself lucky they were scientists and luddites, with no desire to blab about their crazy daughter on the internet. And that I was lucky enough to grow up before Facebook."[4]

Then I looked for a way to justify my own writing about my kids, looking around for what could set me apart. I settled on my own neurodivergence:

Does my own disability shift the genre, though? Bend it, just enough, to make it palatable? I don't know, not yet. I don't think most of these other parents really set out to exploit their children. I think most genuinely struggled, and writing eased their pain. But I do think it's harder to relate to your kid's disabled experience when you aren't disabled yourself.

It is true that I have a different perspective on parenting neurodivergent kids because I grew up ND too. But my words are unfair to neurotypical parent-writers who take care in their writing, such as Chung. In wrestling with my own fear that I was exploiting my ND kids, I patted myself on the back for being a neurodivergent parent, as though that gave me a free pass in my writing. (It didn't.)

* * *

Over the years, I have made plenty of mistakes. But the more I wrote about my kids, the more I learned to do things right. I ended up creating a code of writing ethics to keep my kids safe when I, their parent, write about them.

> *Rule #1: Your kid is the hero of the story.* Write only about the times your children are at their best, their most beautiful. Don't lay out your kids' worst moments for the world to consume. If you need to complain about your kids, pick up the phone and call a friend—we all need support, and there is nothing wrong with that. But those complaints should stay private. In your writing, let your love and admiration for your kids shine through. If your love and admiration don't shine through, do not write about your kids.

> *Rule #2: Keep your kids' faces off the internet.* Don't be fooled by privacy settings on social media—those protect nothing in the age of screenshots. Plus, they're breached and changed so frequently that you never know what's actually private from month to month. The internet is forever, and a kid's privacy is gone the first time you post a photo. I didn't post my first photo of my kids until the eldest was a teenager and gave me

permission, after a long talk about what it means to have your face on the internet. This was around the same time that we, their parents, started talking to them about their own social media accounts and posting responsibly. The least we as parents can do is post responsibly, too.

Rule #3: Keep your kids' names out of your writing. As I said in Rule #2, content posted on the internet lasts forever. We do not want our kids to be searchable by name, at least not because of our writing (and not at all if we can help it), until they're ready to enter public life.

Rule #4: Be vague in order to keep your kids safe. Avoid giving school details, for example. Avoid giving day-to-day details at all, if you can help it, such as the time of school pickup and drop-off. Don't say "6 A.M.," just say "early." I know this might seem counterintuitive because you're also writing about their lives, but the point of this rule is to keep your kids safe.

Rule #5: Tell your own story. This rule gets to the heart of why people write about their kids in the first place. I'm very protective of children—as are most humans—especially neurodivergent children. And too often, when parents write about their kids, they are telling the kid's story. Rather than writing a story about themselves, in which their kid happens to be a marvelous hero, the parent writes a story that belongs to the kid, one that may be embarrassing or otherwise private. Ask yourself: Am I writing to figure out more about me and my life and the world? Does this story belong to me? If the answers are no, then don't write the story.

Rule #6: Don't complain about your kids. If you write woe-is-I stories about how hard it is to be a parent, there are repercussions. If your kid is neurodivergent and you complain about how hard it is to parent them, you are not only harming your relationship with your kid, but you are also feeding into the already bloated stereotype that neurodivergent people, and all disabled people, are a drag on society. Imagine what your readers might think: *Not even their own parents want to take care of them.* Vent in private; praise in your writing.

Rule #7: Put safeties in place. Have your coparent or someone close to your family read your writing. And, if they're old enough, have your children do so, too. If you're ashamed or afraid to let your family read what you wrote about your kids, ask yourself why. Are you treating your kids with kindness, respect, and gratitude? If so, then those things will shine through.

Rule #8: If you are uncertain about writing about your kids, don't write about your kids. If you are writing a story and wondering whether to put something in or leave it out, leave it out. The uncertainty itself is the answer. Only write about your kids if you are certain that you can do it right.

Every day, I do my best to follow these rules.

* * *

I do a lot of writing in my private notebooks. I write about the marvelous things my kids do. I write about the painful things they live through because our world doesn't make space for people who are different. Writing about their lives helps me figure out how to help them better in the future.

So, when something difficult happens, first I describe the event as clearly as possible, along with how I reacted and how the event made me feel. Everything, from start to finish. When I'm done, I let a few days pass. Then, I reread the story and write reflections. Were my reactions overreactions? (Usually not.) Should I have done something differently? (Sometimes yes.)

In this way, my notebooks help me spot patterns so that I can do better in similar future situations. As my kids have grown older, I've realized that the patterns I spotted in their lives were patterns that I could point to in my own childhood. I realized that my kids were going through experiences similar to those that I went through as a child. And most importantly, I realized that, because of my own childhood experiences, I knew better how to help them. These realizations all came to a head on one particularly awful day at our neighborhood pool when my younger kid was tossed off the swim team for, as they told me, needing too much "individual attention"— a bogeyman for parents of neurodivergent kids. I felt so lost that day, but the one thing I could hold onto was that I'd been where he was decades before, many times before, and I knew the path we would need to walk. I also knew what words to say to make sure my kid knew that he was loved, valued, and good.

Although I began this writing journey in 2018 and I was diagnosed with bipolar disorder in my early twenties, I wasn't diagnosed with autism until 2020. Being autistic made so much sense. My kids were already diagnosed with attention deficit hyperactivity disorder and autism (sometimes called AuDHD). I could see, clearly, that we are all perfectly autistic. We make sense to each other.

To write this book, I researched our collective past by digging through records of past school administrative meetings, parent-teacher conferences, and behavior notes sent home. As

I sifted through old documents, I realized once again that I always underestimate how much it hurts to write about the mistreatment of my children and of myself as a young child. But the work was important. Researching and writing this book about parenting neurodivergent children helped me become a better parent. I hope that this book, which I wrote for all parents of neurodivergent kids, for anyone who lives or works with neurodivergent kids, and for anyone who loves them, will help you too.

YOUR KID BELONGS HERE

Introduction

This book is for all parents who want to better guide their neurodivergent kids through a world that wasn't made for neurodiversity. In each chapter, we will tackle the different challenges that kids like ours face in order to learn how to help them handle these challenges and thrive along the way. I define neurodiversity as normal variations in human neurological function—emphasis on *normal*. Neurodivergent (ND) refers to a person whose neurological function varies from the typical.

I am a neurodivergent—bipolar-autistic—mother of two neurodivergent kids. Raising them in a neurotypical world that rarely makes space for us caused me to look back to my own childhood, when I was often misunderstood and mistreated by kids, adults, and family. I am also a disability studies scholar and a professor of twenty years with both a law degree and a doctorate in rhetoric, which means I am an expert in how public discourse influences law and policy, in particular related to mental health and neurodiversity.

My expertise shapes the structure of the book. In each chapter, you will find stories of my childhood, adulthood, and parenthood. You will also find interviews with other parents of neurodivergent kids who were willing to share their stories, too. I pair these stories with the latest research on neurodivergence, such as anxiety, masking, stimming, meltdowns, school struggles, bullying, and more. Then, I bring together the stories and research to advise our work as parents.

I started working as a neurodiversity writer and advocate after leaving my full-time higher education career. For ten years, I worked in academia while hiding my bipolar diagnosis for fear of being fired. On the day I was promoted, I realized I couldn't stay in hiding any longer because it took too much of a toll on my mental health.[1] So I quit my job, went public with my diagnosis, and started writing a column on mental illness and disability.[2] I went from living the life of a professor to the life of a neurodiversity advocate.

Meanwhile, I gave birth to two kids within two years. For years, I did not know my kids were neurodivergent. So long as we were at home, everything was *normal*. But when my kids grew older and stepped outside the home to attend school, play sports, or go to camps, they suffered. Other kids bullied them. They were kicked off of teams by impatient adults. Adults who should have cared for them didn't protect them or give them the help they needed to thrive. (Indeed, research shows that ND kids are frequently bullied and that adults ignore and even enable this bullying.)[3] Worse, many of these adults punished them for being different. Eventually, they were diagnosed with both attention deficit hyperactivity disorder (ADHD) and autism.

As I fought to protect my children, I felt a sense of familiarity because their experiences were eerily like my own when I was young. As I held my crying child, memories came rushing back of how poorly I was treated in my own life. I took those awful memories and made a vow: I would protect my kids the way I should have been protected, and I would give them the unconditional love and support I should have been given.

Soon after my kids were diagnosed, I was diagnosed with autism myself. I am part of an epidemic of late-diagnosed autistic women who suffered under the sexist and narrow-minded diagnostic methods that persist even today, what researchers call the "lost generation."[4] As my kids grew from toddlers to middle schoolers, I learned that the world has little space for ND kids like them or the kid I once was. Or, for that matter, the adult I am now.

One thing that helped me through these difficult years was that my kids' challenges and strengths—and the world's reactions to them—are deeply familiar to me. Every time a coach has bellowed at one of my kids, I didn't just empathize with their terror or humiliation. No, I felt the frozen-in-place-horror first-hand. The experiences uncorked memories I'd locked down decades ago. Just like my kids, I was impulsive and distracted in gym class. I was overstimulated by raucous chaos and struggled to deal with dysregulated emotions. Like them, when a teacher scolded and humiliated me, I shut down.

My children's suffering at the hands of narrow-minded adults and unkind children reminded me of my own early days of nearly being expelled from first grade because of an intolerant teacher and bad reactions to ADHD medications, which is common in kids with autism. Like them, I had trouble at stressful swim meets and other sporting events, and I had difficulty understanding the humor of my peers, so I was perpetually the butt of jokes. Neurodivergent children are far more likely to be bullied in school; autistic middle and high school students are victims of bullying at a rate of 67 percent compared to the neurotypical student rate of 20 percent.[5] My family has lived that statistic.

Today, I am still digging out of the trauma that I suffered as a child, a young adult, and a woman in my twenties. Autism and other neurodivergences make people vulnerable not only to bullying but also to sexual assault and domestic violence, both of which I experienced. My parents loved me, but they didn't know how to help me. They thought that forcing me to conform would be best. Despite their good intentions, they taught me to doubt myself by trampling my emotional and bodily boundaries, common among parents of ND kids. Indeed, as I've parented my own kids and learned more and more about what they need, I can see how I, too, trampled their boundaries and caused harm. I forced them to wear uncomfortable clothes, to eat foods that repelled them, to do activities they hated. What the research shows is this: when we take away our children's autonomy, they stop trusting us, and they stop trusting themselves. Both are tragedies. All I can do now is work hard to make up for these failures.

Today, I draw from my childhood experiences as a source of strength. I know what harmed me as a child. I know how I should have been treated by the adults who were supposed to keep me safe. When I needed patience, silence, or private time, I rarely received it. But now my own children get those things. I also draw on my professional expertise to help me parent better. For example, I don't force my kids to wear itchy clothes or otherwise try to "toughen them up" because I've learned, through my work studying neurodiversity, that this kind of "exposure" doesn't fix anything. It only creates years of trauma for ND kids to deal with.[6]

I know that when you push a kid too hard, they might shut down, and that shutting down is normal and okay. Adults often want answers, right now. Adults want to know what kids are feeling—immediately. These are unreasonable expectations for most kids. For ND kids, they're impossible. Not everyone with the same diagnoses has the same experiences, but my life experiences and life's work have given me a special window into ND kids' lives, and I'm grateful for it.

Most importantly, kids aren't all the same, even if adults wish they were. They come in a beautiful variety. They come like mine, they come like yours, they come like I did, and they come like you did. Some are able to conform to adult expectations better than others, but every one of them is unique. And by asking children to be the same, we hurt all children. We also miss out on the incredible gifts of ND kids. By viewing ND kids as problems to be solved or diagnoses to be cured, our society fails to see the strengths and talents of these children and of the adults they will become.

THE WORLD WILL NOT BEND
FOR OUR CHILDREN

When my older son was six, the summer before first grade, I had his reading skills evaluated by a speech and language pathologist because I was concerned about his progress in school. After the evaluation, the SLP gave me her report: language acquisition disorder, what is colloquially called dyslexia.

His vocabulary was off the charts. His ability to use words in a sentence and define them was excellent. But his ability to read and write words was dramatically weaker than these other skills. The SLP told me that the wide gulf between his abilities would be incredibly frustrating for him—as it would be for anybody. My son needed support to bring those skills into alignment.

Armed with her written evaluation, I approached his public school for help. After many, often adversarial meetings, his school refused to provide the extra help he needed. Why? Because he wasn't failing his classes. He had a steady stream of mediocre report cards that showed, apparently, that he was doing adequately in school. (An "adequate" education is all that schools are required to provide, and what adequate means is often not adequate at all.)[7]

After the meeting, I called my husband in tears. "Who cares what his grades are? He can't read."

My kid seemed happy enough at his school, though, so we kept him enrolled. Then we paid the private SLP breathtaking—yet appropriate—sums to teach our son how to read and write. (Insurance often doesn't cover the help of therapists like SLPs.) With her help, he made great strides, but reading and writing were still an immense challenge, and he needed help beyond the private sessions. He needed help in school itself.

At the beginning of second grade, we transferred our two kids to the only private school in our small town, hoping for better reading support for our older son. We struck gold: Our son's second-grade teacher was supportive and kind, working closely with him on his language skills and accommodating him in all of his subjects. But the relief we felt was short-lived. Our younger son, who was just starting kindergarten, was soon having a hard time with his teacher.

One day, out of the blue, his kindergarten teacher called us in for a meeting. She started with words I will never forget. "I've been teaching for thirty years," she said. "And I've never had such a difficult student. I'm at the end of my rope with him."

Her words crushed me. What did it mean that in thirty years of teaching, no student had ever been as difficult as my son? Did it mean that when she saw him, she resented him? Did "end of my rope" mean she'd given up on him?

I wondered, coldness washing over me, *Is my son safe in this woman's care?*

My husband asked her to describe what our son did that bothered her so much.

"He hides under the table," she revealed, as though this behavior were the equivalent of smoking meth on the playground.

Taking in her austere face and rigid demeanor, I thought, *I would hide too.*

Later that fall, the SLP—whom my older son continued to work with—gave me an update on his progress. At the end of our meeting, she said to me gently, "I think you should have him evaluated for ADHD." Attention deficit hyperactivity disorder is a developmental disorder that can affect a person's ability to concentrate, plan, and execute multistep tasks and to focus on their work.

I felt rattled by her revelation, but I took her advice and began the process of evaluating both of my sons for ADHD. There were so many appointments—the pediatrician first, then the psychologists for days of testing while I sat in the waiting room trying to keep up with work on my laptop. It didn't occur to me at the time that the diagnostic process for ND people is overly burdensome. I can see it now, though, having gone through it three times with them. Testing not only costs thousands of dollars, but it also takes an immense amount of time out of an adult's working life. Plus, finding psychologists who do testing is difficult, and most have long wait lists.[8] When all of the testing was through, both of my kids were diagnosed with ADHD and autism. We were lucky—we could afford psychological testing for our children and, later, for me.

Because testing is so burdensome, many, if not most, families can't get their kids tested at all. Barriers to testing are worse for Black children, poor children, and children of immigrant families.[9] And without testing, ND kids can't get support in school. As a consequence, adults who went undiagnosed in childhood struggle with self-identity, anxiety, depression, grief, and even suicide. Fortunately, self-diagnosis tools are helpful and valid for adults seeking to understand their own neurodivergent identities.[10] (I encourage you to investigate them. Neurodivergences are genetic, after all.)

The list of diagnoses of my kids and me don't tell the real story. The story has always been about a world that only sees ND people as problems to be solved—or, worse, erased altogether. When faced with frustrated or angry adults, my older son would freeze, unable to speak. My younger son literally took cover. I would do the same as a child, and when I grew older, I would erupt and fight back.

Being a child is wildly unfair. Grown-ups expect children to be little adults. But that's not possible. Kids' memories don't work like adults' do, and they can't express themselves like an adult can—telling linear stories recounted with precision. We expect kids to sit still and silently, for hours, essentially dissociating themselves from their bodies. Sure, some kids are reserved. But others are exuberant. And there should be room for all of them.

During that meeting with the kindergarten teacher, it became apparent that she didn't bother to understand my kid. After she told us he kept hiding under his desk, I said, "Did you ask him why he's hiding?"

Miffed, the teacher said, "Well, no."

Later in the conference, she told us, "I can't make him do the things the students are supposed to do."

I thought, *Why would you want to make anyone do anything?*

You don't make people you love do things. And you don't force children to do things. You work together, you explain, and you teach.

That day was all the more awful because I knew a secret: how much my kid wanted to please this teacher. He told me so all the time. "I want to make her happy, Mommy." He just didn't know how.

Later that day, back at home, I asked my son, "Why do you hide under your desk at school sometimes?"

He said, "I get worried."

Tell me, honestly: While a pandemic raged, while our Capitol was stormed, while fires burn and earthquakes devastate, while wars tear countries and the world apart, while police brutality puts a new tragic headline in the news every week, while, as I finish this introduction, government changes threaten the very thin protections in place for people like me and my children, and yours, wouldn't you hide under your desk if you could?

The world is *worrisome.*

Things were not, are not, hard for me because my kids are hard. No. Things are hard for me as a parent because the world makes things *impossible* for my kids. My kids are perfectly imperfect—in that way, they're like all kids. And like many parents of ND kids, I see the world as an ocean with titanic waves, threatening to drown us, and I'm a small ship holding us afloat. Yes, I'm tired. But never, ever because of them.

I know that this world will not bend for my children. But I will not let my ugly childhood past repeat itself. I will do whatever it takes to make sure my kids' journey is better than mine was. I will not force my kids to contort themselves into someone else's conception of "normal" as I was pushed to do. I will not trample their boundaries, but instead, I will teach them how to set healthy ones and insist that others respect them.

With this book, I hope to show all parents that they are not alone, that their fears are normal, and that the challenges that they face as parents are, in the end, surmountable.

WHO IS THIS BOOK FOR?

I wrote this book for *all* parents of neurodivergent children and also for parents whose kids struggle with fitting in or who do things a little differently. After all, you don't have to have a formal diagnosis to feel alienated from our social norms. This book is also for anyone interested in the social and cultural forces at play at the intersection of neurodiversity and parenthood.

I wrote this book for every parent who has felt like a misfit or failure, who wasn't sure that they had what it takes to parent their kid, or who believed that they were unprepared, unfit, or unworthy. I wrote it for every parent who suffered as a child and whose memories of that suffering haunt them every day as they swear that they won't make the same mistakes or pass down legacies of pain and hurt. To those parents, I say, *You can break those cycles.*

Parenting is already a lonely endeavor in our society, where most of us live with our kids in our isolated homes, often flung far from family or friends. Or maybe those family and friends are too overworked or busy to help. Every parent must regularly fight against loneliness, yes, but parenting a child who is marginalized by schools, clubs, camps, and teams can make it nearly impossible for a parent to find community. Communities are stripped from you, just as they're stripped from your child. To you, I say, *You are not alone.*

I'm writing for every parent of ND kids who has wanted to bend the world in half because of how it has mistreated their children. Who wanted to scream and yell at teachers and coaches and camp counselors for the petty and not-so-petty cruelties visited on their children. Who don't want a seat at the table for their kids but rather want to smash that table to pieces and build a new one.

And last, I'm writing this book for every scared kid who wanted to hide under their desk at school, or in the shadowed corner of the school dance they were forced to attend, or behind the driver of the school bus hoping for safety from bullies. That kid was me. And it might be yours. They deserve our protection, and we can give it to them.

SCARCITY

Two interlocking principles guide this book. The first is our "culture of scarcity,"[11] the idea that there is not enough of a resource to go around, such as funds for education. The second is the concept of "social norms," which are the shared rules of behavior that a group of people adhere to. Social norms are harmful when they punish certain people for behavior simply because it appears strange. These two principles are large in scale and institutional and help us better understand what causes the harm that our ND kids experience. Understanding the bigger picture helps us be better advocates for our children.

In a "culture of scarcity," a concept popularized by psychologist Brené Brown, people believe that there is not enough of a resource to go around—even when there is. Brown calls this "The Never-Enough Problem."[12] The scarcity we encounter might not feel like false scarcity in our day-to-day lives. It can seem quite real. Let me explain.

I hear about many heartbreaking arguments from school administrators, other parents, coaches, and more about how ND kids are a "drain" on resources. In this context, "resources" means money and what that money represents. Rather than viewing ND kids as simply another user of a resource, other parents, teachers, and coaches resent ND kids. But some basic questions reveal how the painful "drain" argument is culturally constructed: Who decided how we allocate resources? Why does a school, camp, or club choose to spend their resources the way they do? Why are resources scarce in the first place? The answers have little to do with whether there are adequate resources and a whole lot to do with how those with institutional power choose to dole them out.

In a culture of scarcity, ND families are pitted against the gatekeepers of resources, such as schools, and against other parents who want to make sure their neurotypical kids get a "fair share." Resources such as schooling, camps, and so forth are supposed to be open to all, not just because it's the right thing to do but because it's the law. The problem is, far too often, ND kids do not receive the resources they need to thrive. For example, I chose to homeschool my children after eventually trying four—four!—different schools. These schools, both public and private, didn't have the resources to meet my kids' basic educational and safety needs. At one private school, an "exceptional children" (EC) teacher told me that she was overworked and overwhelmed and wouldn't be able to adequately support my kids. (I deeply appreciated her candor.) At a public school, the EC teacher told me, in private, that the school would not be able to meet the needs of my kids because of allocation of funds. (Once again, a teacher's honesty was lifesaving.) But whose fault is it that schools and sports teams fail to provide resources to ND kids? Whose fault is it that parents of neurotypical kids believe that ND kids steal all of the attention?

Even though I've had terrible experiences with individual teachers, coaches, and other kids who have harmed my kids, and I've taken steps to mitigate that harm, I've rarely blamed the organizations themselves. Instead, my training has taught me to look at issues such as a scarcity at the societal and cultural level. I ask, "What are the larger forces at play that cause pain to one individual child?" I ask, "Why is there scarcity in the first place when we live in a culture of such wealth?"

You can draw a connection from one vote in Congress or one ruling in a court all the way down to my singular child being unfairly suspended from school because he finally defended himself against a bully. When I say "connection," I am not talking about a butterfly effect. I am talking about a direct line from large-scale policy decisions to our everyday lives. Decisions made by politicians and judges who are far removed from children deprive them of resources. Even as I've been writing this introduction, I received an email from our public school district that it is slashing jobs yet again, and I tried to imagine the frustration that the administrators and teachers must feel when facing even more financial cuts.

Schools struggle with a lack of experienced teachers and low pay because of budgets set by distant politicians. Therapists (occupational, speech, and so on) struggle with undercutting of their fees by for-profit insurance companies and Medicaid, and many, if not most, opt not to accept insurance at all. Camps and sports teams, especially ones supported by local governments, can't find experienced adults who are willing to accept the pay they offer or who are willing to volunteer. College admission tests are run by for-profit organizations whose bottom lines rely upon an illusion of reliability, and so they block ND kids from accommodations that appear like "getting a leg up."

The problem is that the connections between institutional forces and our everyday experiences can be hard to see. We see the individual teachers and coaches who harm our kids, and we should definitely hold them, their supervisors, and their institutions accountable. But we must also understand why these bad things keep happening.

My favorite metaphor for how scarcity affects the lives of ND families is an ancient gladiator pit. ND families are tossed in a pit to fight against schools and teachers; against camps and sports teams; against college admission tests; against occupational therapists, psychologists, and social workers; and against other parents who are convinced that our kids steal resources from their own. Down in the pit, our culture of scarcity turns us into enemies forced to fight each other over what we believe are finite resources.

But the truth is that we battle over a *false* scarcity of resources, one deliberately created by politicians and lobbyists who divert money away from ND and other disabled children and toward their private interests. Continuing with my metaphor, the people holding the purse strings sit in upper echelons of the Colosseum, bored with the battle below, content in their wealth, knowing their power remains intact so long as we, the gladiators, continue to fight one another and ignore where the real problems lie.

When you consider how much ND families must fight for the resources we need, it becomes easier to see how we have, all of us, been set up to lose in a game of divide and conquer. For example, after (metaphorically) fighting with schools, my family finally pulled out of schools altogether in order to homeschool. We lost our battle in the pit. But who won when my kids stayed home? The schools? Or the policymakers who have one less ND kid to educate?

Fortunately, there are other types of advocates holding policymakers' feet to the fire to bring about change. That is not the work I do as a writer. But a large part of solving a problem is spreading the knowledge that it exists in the first place. Once again, I am not excusing the harm our children suffered in schools, camps, or teams. We must still hold these organizations accountable. But for real change to come, it must come from a place far higher than our local middle schools or soccer teams.

SOCIAL NORMS

As disability studies scholar Lennard J. Davis has written, "We live in a world of norms."[13] Social norms are the shared, often invisible, rules of behavior that a group of people adhere to. Groups creates social norms based on what traits and behaviors are considered "normal." Norms can be good: They encourage us not to punch someone on the street or steal cars. But social norms can also cause harm because, if you do not meet "normal" social expectations, you are punished. The very existence of norms creates, as Davis puts it, "deviations and extremes."[14] In the context of disabilities/neurodiversity, because our society operates under a system of norms, then disabled/neurodivergent people are, as Davis puts it, "deviants."[15] Put simply, if you are neurodivergent, then you are made wrong—a deviation from the norm.[16]

Norms are not neutral; rather, they are a method of determining who is better than another and how. As Davis explains, we use social norms to "rank our intelligence, our cholesterol level, our weight, height, sex drive, bodily dimensions along some conceptual line from subnormal to above-average."[17] Thus, in reality, "norms" aren't about averages but rather a way to place more value on some people and less value on others. For example, Davis writes, "Although high intelligence in a normal distribution would simply be an extreme, under a ranked system it would become the highest ranked trait."[18] The norm and the ranking of the ideal tell us how we *should* be, which is a social requirement, not a suggestion. If you stray from the "normal ideal" (a phrase that sounds antithetical but is how norms work in practice), then you are marginalized and victimized.

Neurotypical social norms are the norms that harm our neurodivergent kids. In his book *Normal Sucks*, neurodivergent author and activist Jonathan Mooney demonstrates how the concept of "normal" hurt him as a child.[19] After years of negative experiences in school because of his undiagnosed learning disabilities, Mooney writes that, at age ten, "I knew people thought something was *wrong* with me."[20] After his diagnosis with language-based learning disabilities and ADHD, he asked his mother, "Am I normal?" Even as a child, Mooney knew that he "had crossed that invisible line between the *normal* and the *not normal*, which we all know is there."

The harm that ND people face is called *ableism*, which is discrimination against disabled people, including ND people, on the basis of their disability or neurodivergence. Ableism permeates the fabric of our society; even neurodivergent people are susceptible to it. Neurodivergent kids and adults experience *internalized ableism*. Internalized ableism can cause ND people to mistreat other ND people and feel self-loathing. Internalized ableism is both sneaky and devastating. When a child is punished for having needs that are beyond the norm, they learn (wrongly) that their needs aren't important and to ignore them. They end up doing whatever it takes to avoid punishment in the future. For ND kids, ignoring their own needs in order to avoid punishment teaches them to hate being neurodivergent (because it causes punishment) and to suppress ("mask") their neurological differences in order to appear neurotypical.

I developed this self-loathing as an undiagnosed autistic kid when it became clear that I couldn't adhere to social norms. When I was young, I learned from adults, and later my peers, that everything about myself was (is) simply wrong. Many of these adults loved me, such as my parents and others who only wanted what was best for me. But our ableist social norms convinced them that the best way to raise me was to make me as neurotypical as possible.

It's taken years of therapy to uncover the wounds caused by my belief in my own wrongness: that I talk too much, that I lack social skills, that I'm not social enough, that I don't have enough friends. These criticisms started when I was young, but they continued into adulthood, both from outsiders and from a self-critical voice inside my own head.

Ableism is the voice that says, "Is my neurodivergent life valuable if I merely live a *normal* life?" And worse, "Is my neurodivergent life valuable if I *drain* resources, rather than contribute?" The answer, of course, is that every life is valuable. Every ND person deserves to be loved, educated, and cared for. There is no such thing as a "drain" on resources. The notion of a "drain" is a lie created by those who let us battle it out in the gladiator pit while they hold the purse strings. Our society has resources, and we are supposed to use them to care for the members of our society. That's literally what it means to live together in a society. Our ND children deserve everything that neurotypical children receive. They are not a burden.

LIMITATIONS OF THIS BOOK

This book necessarily has limitations. First, I am a white, cisgender woman in a heterosexual marriage. Although there are a higher number of queer people among autistics than among neurotypicals,[21] and I am indeed one of these queer people among autistics, being in a long-term heterosexual marriage gives me many social benefits. I also have financial resources that many people do not have, including a stable income and good health insurance. My family's resources enable me to get professional psychological testing for me and my family and give us access to excellent mental health care.

Neurodivergent people of color are, for many reasons, under-represented in the research literature. Their unique experiences are understudied and misunderstood by professionals. One reason is that people of color face barriers to diagnoses because, as autistic Black author and advocate Kala Allen Omeiza points out, "most healthcare systems across the world overlook symptoms of autism that aren't presented as the standard clinical and research norm [that word again] which is currently Western white males."[22] Therefore, studies of groups of autistic people, ADHDers, or people with anxiety disorders will necessarily have fewer people of color. I have done my best to bring in the voices of Black and other racially and ethnically marginalized autistic people.

Furthermore, stories by ND people of color are not given the same airtime that publishers, magazines, and TV and film studios give to white neurodivergent stories. My story is a white woman's story. After you finish this book, I encourage you to read stories, whether novels or nonfiction, by neurodivergent Black writers,[23] Asian American writers,[24] Latinx writers,[25] Indigenous writers[26]—by *all* of the writers whose racial and ethnic diversity creates the full meaning of "neurodiversity."

Gender and sex present another challenge. Whenever this book refers to "motherhood" or "mother," I refer to a person who has given birth, whether cis, trans, nonbinary, or gender-queer. When I use the terms "girl" and "woman," I refer to all girls and women, whether cis or trans. If you identify as a mother, you are a mother in the context of this book. The same goes for fathers. Despite my own intentions with gendered language, when I write about neurodiversity research, diagnosis, and treatment, I must rely on scientific research that uses strict gender binaries. That scientists studying neurodiversity continue to lean heavily on a strict binary is ironic given the high rates of gender-fluid and transgender people among neurodivergent people, especially autistic people.[27] This bias in the underlying scientific research presents another limitation to my work.

THE LANGUAGE OF NEURODIVERSITY

How we *talk* about neurodivergent people affects how we *treat* neurodivergent people. For this reason, I'm providing a short guide on the language of neurodiversity.

Neurodiversity. I define neurodiversity as normal variations in human neurological function—emphasis on *normal*. But unlike some other normal human variations (e.g., height), neurodiversity isn't celebrated or even ignored. It is penalized. The word "neurodiversity" is a portmanteau of "neurological diversity," popularized by Australian sociologist Judy Singer back in 1998 in the context of autism.[28] Today its usage has expanded to include the wide variety of neurodivergences in the world, including anxiety, depression, bipolar disorder, post-traumatic stress disorder (PTSD), and brain fog. An individual who has a normal variation in human neurological function can be called "neurodivergent" (shortened to ND in this book). Some neurodivergent people also identify as disabled, and many neurodivergences qualify as disabilities under the Americans with Disabilities Act (ADA), when seeking Social Security benefits, and under the Individuals with Disabilities Education Act (IDEA).

Neurotypical. When referring to a person who is not neurodivergent, you can use various terms. The most common one is "neurotypical" (NT). You might hear the term "abled," which

means how it sounds: not-disabled. A third word you might encounter is "normate," a term coined by disability studies scholar
Rosemarie Garland-Thomson to refer to nondisabled people.[29]

Ableism. Ableism is discrimination against disabled people,
including neurodivergent people, on the basis of their disabil-
ity/neurodivergence. Ableism, like any other form of discrimination, permeates the fabric of our society and is hard to spot
despite its painful effects. Neurodivergent people can also be
ableist through "internalized ableism."

Stigma. I define stigma against neurodivergent people as a
process that creates negative stereotyping and isolation, typically based on the irrational fear of undesirable behavior such
as irresponsibility, instability, or violence. Stigma also works in-
ternally on disabled people, creating feelings of isolation and
shame.[30] The key term here is "irrational." In our shared public
imagination, neurodivergent people are scary and dangerous,
despite the fact that we are no more likely to be violent toward
others than anyone else.[31] For example, if you look at the (irrational) public discourse after any large-scale act of gun violence,
you will see how quick our society is to blame neurodivergent
people for this particular social ill, even if the perpetrator isn't
neurodivergent but rather a white supremacist (e.g., those who
have targeted synagogues and Black churches) or a rabid misog-
ynist (e.g., those who have targeted women scientists or sorori-
ties). But despite how irrational stigma may be, it causes serious harm to neurodivergent people. It tells us that it is shameful
to seek mental health support. It makes us feel isolated and
alone. It causes anxiety, depression, and even death by suicide.

Accommodations and accessibility. "Accommodations" and
"accessibility" are two words that people often think mean
the same thing, but they could not be more different. Ideally,
both accommodations and accessibility are meant to make

our neurotypical world easier for ND people to live in, and, in their best forms, they do. But, as I've written, "Accommodations are not accessibility. Accommodations are special exceptions made for one disabled person who has to jump through lots of hoops to get them." Those hoops include, for example, expensive psychological testing that most families with neurodivergent kids cannot access. On the other hand, "Accessibility is the creation of a space that is hospitable to and usable by disabled people, no hoops required."[32]

But because we live in an inaccessible world, we need accommodations. As I explain, "Accommodations are only necessary because a workplace, a school, or a society creates spaces that are inaccessible to neurodivergent people. When a neurodivergent person encounters an inaccessible space, they inevitably need accommodations."[33] As Andrew Solomon writes in *Far from the Tree: Parents, Children, and the Search for Identity*, "In the vast literature about disability rights, scholars stress the separation between *impairment*, the organic consequence of a condition, and *disability*, the result of social context."[34] In an accessible world, neurodivergent people would still have our impairments, but we would not be disabled by an ableist, neuro-normative environment that puts obstacles in our way.

Masking. "Masking" refers to when ND people hide our neurological and behavioral differences. We hide these differences from neurotypical people and social groups in order to keep ourselves safe and to make neurotypical people feel more comfortable.[35] But neurodivergent masking causes exhaustion, burnout, anxiety, depression, and suicide. In spaces where neurodiversity is accepted, neurodivergent people feel less pressure to mask. But, after a lifetime of masking, it can be hard to stop, especially because we frequently do not realize that we are doing it.[36]

BOOK OVERVIEW

This book contains a preface, which describes how the book came to be; this introduction, which discusses the purpose and audience of the book; and six chapters.

Chapter 1, "The Exclusion of Neurodivergent Kids from Public Life," describes how neurodivergent kids are frequently kept out of schools, camps, teams, and more because of a common refrain: "They require too much individual attention." What I call the "individual attention fallacy" hides the insistence on conformation to irrelevant, overly narrow, ableist social norms. By uncovering this fallacy, we can see that it is ableism, not our children, that is causing the problem, a realization that is both freeing and galvanizing.

Chapter 2, "Previewing, Meltdowns, and Social Policing," addresses emotional expression by neurodivergent kids that our ableist society deems unacceptable. It delves into how these behaviors are actually helpful to ND kids and why they happen in the first place. I discuss social policing, which is one way that social norms against ND kids are enforced in our everyday lives, and the consequences of this policing for both parents and kids. In the end, I talk about how to reject social policing of our children and how to understand and embrace ND behavior.

Chapter 3, "Masking, Treatments, and Affirming Neurodiversity," examines our ableist society's urge to force ND children to comply with "normal" standards of behavior. Neurodivergent kids cope with this pressure by masking or self-stimulatory behavior ("stimming"). But, in neurotypical society, stimming is not socially acceptable. Kids end up suppressing their need to stim, which causes psychological damage, including anxiety, depression, and suicidal thoughts. The chapter also looks at the ways that parents are encouraged to seek treatments that will make ND children seem more neurotypical, believing that the appearance of neurotypicality will make children happier. In the end, the chapter encourages parents to avoid forcing our children to mask their neurodivergences, to push back against ableist social norms, and to find neurodiversity-affirming care for our children.

Chapter 4, "The Medication Double Bind," addresses how ableism pressures parents' decisions about medication and their neurodivergent kids. A double bind is a situation in which a person faces two conflicting demands, usually from some force more powerful than they are. For parents of ND kids, on the one hand, society pressures us to make our kids (seem) more neurotypical. On the other hand, we're pressured to avoid medicating our kids because of the stigma against both medication and our kids' diagnoses. Whatever parents decide, we can't win. To beat the double bind, parents must find professionals whom they trust and should involve their children in the decision-making, creating a plan that works best for them while ignoring stigma and public pressure. (This is not easy.)

Chapter 5, "School Accommodations," talks about the many issues that ND kids and families face with schools: obtaining individualized education programs (IEPs), dealing with how race affects schools' approach to neurodiversity, and twice-exceptional (2E) neurodivergent kids who have both intellectual gifts and support needs, whom schools struggle to accommodate. I address homeschooling and the options that parents have on that front. In the end, decisions about schooling are personal to each kid and to each family, but knowing what options are available will help us make informed decisions.

Chapter 6, "Bullying, Vulnerability, and Trauma," addresses the rampant bullying that neurodivergent kids face, not just from other kids but also from adults. I discuss who is vulnerable and why, bullying in schools, why and how adults victimize children, and what we, as parents, can do to help our children learn to protect themselves.

Thank you for taking this journey with me as we learn together how to be better parents for our ND kids.

CHAPTER 1

The Exclusion of Neurodivergent Kids from Public Life

My mom often tells me that I was a difficult kid to raise. She says that I was stubborn, overly energetic, and prone to meltdowns, all starting at age one and a half.

Because I was such a difficult kid, my mom sought out one of the best child psychiatrists in the country, who happened to practice in the midsize southern town where we lived. What finally sent my mom to the doctor was not something that I had done but rather something that was done to me. At age four, I had been kicked out of our preschool carpool. My mom felt both ashamed and worried.

Years later, when I was in high school, my mom told me the kicked-out-of-carpool story. We were in the kitchen of my childhood home, with its dark wood cabinets and the stained glass window over the sink. I was leaning against the counter while she was cooking. My mom always cooked when her emotions were high—when she was nervous, stressed out, or angry—using every pot in the kitchen like they'd offended her.

When she told me about how a group of moms threw me out of the carpool, I thought the story was hilarious. But my mom wasn't laughing.

"What happened?" I asked.

"They told me you were too disruptive."

I knew the moms who had fired me from the carpool. Acquaintances of my parents, they were our neighbors and people we ran into at local restaurants. And they were the worst snobs. As my mom told me the story, I tried to picture them fifteen years before, with their pinched faces, afraid I would taint their precious offspring with my weirdness. It was easy for me to laugh, though. I was off to a top college in the fall, and my future was bright. At age seventeen, I couldn't understand why my mother still cared about what had happened in preschool.

In the kitchen that day, with four pots on the stove, my mom tried to make me understand. The carpool story wasn't funny to her at all. It was gut-wrenching, the equivalent of a *Mean Girls* rejection from the lunch table—except instead of the Mean Girls rejecting her, they rejected her child.

I didn't get it then, but now that I'm a mom, I do. I realize how devastating it is to have someone attack your kid. The other moms had made mine feel as though there were something inherently wrong with me. When they told my mom that I had to go, they gave her a litany of reasons: I talked too much in the car. I wouldn't sit quietly. I wouldn't stand still in the parking lot but instead bounced around too much. They thought my behavior was so terrible that they didn't want me anymore. I'm sure I did all of the things that the carpool moms complained about. I still have trouble sitting still, and I definitely still talk a lot. And my own kids do those same things today.

When I was four years old and my mom met with the child psychiatrist, she dumped out all of her fears and worries about me. "What's wrong with her?" my mom asked. "How can I fix her?"

The psychiatrist, an extraordinarily calm woman, said, "Your daughter isn't the problem."

"She's not?"

The doctor shook her head. "They made you feel like she is. Don't let them."

"How?" my mother asked. My mom needed something to fix on, a North Star.

Fortunately, the psychiatrist could give her one. She provided my mother with three touchstone questions:

- Did the child put other kids in danger?
- Did she put herself in danger?
- Did she damage property?

According to the psychiatrist, if the answer to all three questions were no, then the punishment I received—banishment— was too severe. Then she uttered words that I want to shout from every mountaintop on planet Earth: "Kids aren't all the same," she said. "And we can't expect them to be. We have to give them some leeway."

Her words were so simple yet so transformative. Without saying it out loud, she was calling for universal inclusion and accessibility.

"What do I do?" my mom asked, frantic with worry.

"Find better people to carpool with," the psychiatrist said.

The psychiatrist's three touchstone questions were likely based on the diagnostic criteria of pediatric conduct disorder, a diagnosis in the American Psychiatric Association's *Diagnostic and Statistical Manual of Mental Disorders* (*DSM*). Conduct disorder "is characterized by a repetitive and persistent pattern of behavior that violates either the rights of others or major age-appropriate societal norms or rules."[1] The main features of conduct disorder are "aggression to people and animals," "destruction of property," "deceitfulness or theft," and "serious violations of rules."[2]

By giving my mother a simplified list of these complex criteria—harm to self, others, or property—the doctor provided the North Star my mother needed, that is, a way to know that her kid was not clinically harmful or dangerous. No, I was just annoying to a group of people who had a low tolerance for anyone who strayed outside their particular set of narrow norms.

The psychiatrist addressed those narrow norms as well. She didn't tell my mom to change me to fit within them. She told her that the carpool's norms were nonsense and to find somewhere else where the norms would fit around me.

This story took on importance as I became a mother to children who have also been excluded from groups, activities, and teams based on irrelevant, narrow social norms. My experience as a child and a daughter has helped me be a better mom. But still, it hasn't been easy. Whenever your child is rejected, it is always painful.

THE SWIM TEAM

It is summertime 2017. I am a grown woman with two sons, ages six and eight. Over the last three years, my kids have been kicked out of many, many places for being different from other kids. The complaints are always the same. Too boisterous. Fidgets. Distractible. Cannot follow directions. Too stubborn. In between the lines, I hear another complaint that few want to say out loud: *Too annoying.*

This morning, I'm watching my younger son, Six, take a private swim lesson. It is early; the air is still cool, and the pool is closed to everyone except us. We're here because Six desperately wants to be on the summer swim team with his brother, Eight. In one week, swim team practice starts, and I am helping Six prepare as much as he can for the new experience. With these swim lessons, we are "previewing," an occupational therapy concept that I define as letting someone know what is coming so that they can prepare for it mentally, especially when, because of how their brains are wired, it is a little harder for them to handle the unexpected than it is for other people.[3] In its best form, previewing is two directional. "Two directional" means that the burden is not only on the ND kid to have their act together in a new situation but also on the neurotypical person or group who will be spending time with the ND kid to make sure that their space is accessible to all kids. In other words, kids shouldn't have to carry the load of the new and scary adventure alone. Instead, the adults in charge of the adventure have a duty to help ND kids find a way to feel safe and enjoy the adventure—like they should do for *all* kids.

This morning, at the swim lesson, I'm previewing the swim team for my kid and also sharing the burden of previewing with the private swim coach. It should not be Six's burden alone to learn about the swim team. He is, after all, only six. During these lessons, the swim coach, one of the young assistants to the head coach, is also getting to know Six. I want her to see where he is brilliant and where he is struggling, what makes him unique and what makes him ordinary. In the end, the coach will see that he is just another six-year-old who wants to join the summer swim team. After two weeks of lessons, she will know him and hopefully care about him. Once swim team starts, she will be his coach, and he will be at her mercy.

I sit on a pool chair, partially reclined, and watch the coach and my kid move around the pool. The swim coach is a young white woman in her early twenties; my son is scrawny and tall, with startlingly pale skin and short, light-blond hair. Their bodies leave a rolling wake as the coach tugs the kickboard my kid clings to. Outwardly, I appear calm, but I am not. Watching them carefully, the coach and my son, I worry that she will get impatient with him and that, in her impatience, she will be cruel. It has happened too many times in the past.

For Six, learning how to swim is not the problem. Six can swim fine. These lessons are about learning how to be on the team: how to listen to a coach, how to follow directions, how to keep his goggles on, how to keep his head above water when the coach is talking, how to stay in the proper lane, and how to do all of the other things that coaches expect children to know how to do, *innately*, in order to participate in group activities. But my kid struggles with how to do these sorts of things innately. He will sometimes forget what you tell him to do shortly after you do so. And he is aware that he forgets. Six is young, but he is very smart, and he knows that he is different. So we're here, preparing for swim team, making sure that Six can do the things the coaches ask.

In retrospect, I can see that I really hired the coach to teach my kid how to avoid being annoying, the mortal sin of a neuro-divergent child. At the time, I wouldn't have been able to put words to this underlying fear. Just like every mom, I want people to like my kids. But my kids tend to evoke strong opinions in adults. That's the thing about being different. You're either different good or different bad. There's rarely a middle ground.

As I watch Six's swim lesson, I'm on edge. Over and over, I hold myself back from intervening in Six's behavior. I'm worried because Six is talking. A lot. Then, when he gets excited about something he's saying, he stops his strokes. He chatters; he fiddles with the kickboard; he bounces up and down on the pool floor. He is acting "distractible," a word I detest, one that is used to describe a particular poor behavior: a failure to give *undivided attention*. Giving adults undivided attention is a moral imperative for children in neurotypical society.

As Six works on his flutter kick with the kickboard, he is explaining his current favorite physics concepts, things like electromagnetic pulses and gravity. He talks and he talks, thrilled to have someone who will listen to his ideas. His ideas are gorgeous. But I know not everyone can see their beauty. Many would prefer that he just shut up because he talks too much. *Different-bad.*

But I don't intervene. I squeeze the edges of the lounge chair, the bolts that secure the metal tubes biting my palms. I think, *If she's a good swim coach, she will know what to do*. After all, he's just talking. He's not doing anything wrong. But, when you're a parent, the urge to encourage your kid to act like the socially constructed model of a normal kid can be overwhelming. This feeling is especially strong when you were once a ND kid yourself and you know what kind of social punishment your kid will face for being different. But, fortunately, I recognize my urge for what it is—internalized ableism—and try to ignore it. Ableism, which is discrimination against disabled people, permeates everything and everyone, including disabled/neurodivergent people ourselves.

I tell myself that Six is allowed to talk during his private swim lesson. He is a human person with feelings and thoughts, and he gets to share them, just like anyone else. Indeed, autistic author and advocate Pete Wharmby urges adults to listen while autistic children talk about their special interests to help them thrive and feel loved and appreciated.[4] Wharmby explains how autistic people's intense special interests are good things for both children and society at large but that neurotypical society often sees these interests as unhealthy obsessions.[5] Neurodivergent and autistic obsession is the reason that I'm writing this book. It revolutionized the gentle care of farm animals (Temple Grandin). It ignited a new environmental movement (Greta Thunberg).

According to my father, I was much like Six when I was starting swim team. At Six's age, my dad had to find coaches who wouldn't get annoyed with me. It was hard, but he did find them. "Once," my dad said, "there was this swim coach, and you stood there, and you were six, and you told him just how the world was. And the coach listened to you talk (and talk), and then he said, 'Katie, that's amazing.'" I recognized in my father's story something that I've felt, too. There's a special joy when another adult sees my kid for who he is and not for what he fails to do.

I've paid for private swim lessons for another reason: so that Six can learn under the very best conditions for Six. The pool is quiet and free of chaos. He has one-on-one time with a coach. And most importantly, during the swim lessons, the coach must bend around Six. After all, Six must bend all the time. I might let him fidget when he is with me, but when he is at school, he gets punished for being too wiggly, or for sharing his ideas when he is not supposed to, or for reading books when he's supposed to be standing in line for lunch. For most of his life, he must try hard to be something other than himself. (Because of the constant punishment he received at school, we started homeschooling during third grade, and he has flourished.)

I have spent my entire life trying to bend to irrational and sometimes impossible social norms, and this bending frequently harmed my mental health. I've learned a word for it now: "masking," when a neurodivergent person hides their neurodivergent traits to appease neurotypical norms. But for most of my life,

I didn't have that word, and I didn't know how much harm I was causing by squishing myself into a tiny neurotypical box. I never want my children to have to mask. I want them to be gloriously themselves.

Here, early in the morning at this pool, I have ensured that my child does not have to bend. I want him to have the confidence that I once had when I was young, before slamming into neurotypical expectations. I will do anything to make sure he is able to hold onto his confidence, even if he doesn't learn to be the best swimmer on the team. I don't even "redirect"—interrupt him when he's going off track and urge him to be quiet so that he can learn what another person might think is appropriate for him to learn. Instead, I let the lesson flow. I don't care if he wins blue ribbons so long as his spirit remains intact.

The coach gives a command, and Six says, "Sure!" He is cheerful and compliant. He wants to make the coach happy. But when she asks an open-ended question, he launches into an exposition about water pressure and depth. That's when I realize that I'm not sure she knows that he just turned six. Although he is as skinny as a noodle, he is tall, like me, physically appearing older than he is. His vocabulary is exorbitant, so his intellectual age seems older, too. He could easily pass for eight or even nine if you only took into account his body and his intelligence. But like many neurodivergent children, he is socially younger than his age, which can be confusing to people who don't take the time to get to know him.

Then, from my pool chair, I hear a subtle change in the tone of the coach's voice. There is impatience, edging toward something worse, like anger. Leaning forward, I watch closely for the moment when the tone crosses that important line. I will allow some impatience. I will not allow meanness. I start keeping count: Six has said "I'm sorry" to her no fewer than ten times. I prepare myself to stand and end the lesson.

Last summer, Six could not even swim across the pool. By the end of the summer, he was launching himself off of the diving board into the deep end like he had been doing it forever. His father and I don't know why he decided to start swimming, except that he did. Once Six decides he wants to do something, he will do it. The inverse is also true. Now, the coach is trying to teach Six how to do side-breathing, but he's struggling with putting his ear in the water.

"It's easy," the coach says, demonstrating. "Just do it like this." She tilts her head to the side until her ear is submerged in the water.

So many neurotypical people take for granted that something is easy when, for neurodivergent people, it isn't easy at all. Concerts, nightclubs, large dinner parties, and other "clangy" events, as my family calls them, are awful. As are certain physical sensations, like itchy clothes tags. If you're a child who struggles to advocate for yourself, how do you explain that it hurts to have water rush into your ear like a fire hose?

Six shakes his head and tries to make her understand. "Easy means easy. Hard means hard. This is hard."

The coach looks confounded.

Six says again, "Like I said. Easy means easy." Then, suddenly, he starts to cry. "Side-breathing puts sixty pounds of pressure on me."

Well, I think. *That doesn't sound easy at all.*

"Just try again," the coach insists, with frustration in her voice.

He says, through tears, "Quit bossing me around."

Despite his tears, I hold back, waiting for the response.

Now, years later, I know that I shouldn't have held back. My children should never have to cry alone to a stranger. Ever.

At Six's words and tears, the coach laughs kindly, breaking the tension that was permeating the pool, and replies, "But that's my job." After Six cries with fear and frustration, struggling under the pressure to do things her way, the coach's annoyance with him disappears. My son has broken down and yielded to her authority. She couldn't deal with his ability to stand up for himself. Six's tears, a show of weakness in the face of her (supposed) superior strength, have finally put her at ease.

Now I know what it looks like to collaborate with a child rather than force them to do something painful or scary. I had to learn it the hard way, after making many mistakes where I pushed my kids around to force them to *respect my authority*. But what I've learned is that they didn't respect me, they feared me. Their tears weren't a sign of sadness but of hopelessness. Of giving up.

Only later did I find out how much the water hurt Six's ears, but he didn't know how to express it in a way that made sense to the coach. The water didn't sting or burn. He felt the pressure on his eardrum, and it squeezed until it felt like "sixty pounds of pressure." Collaborating with a child requires us to listen to how they express themselves, whatever that method is. And most importantly, to believe them.

Because I didn't know better, I left Six alone in the pool with the swim coach instead of intervening on his behalf. When we spoke in private, Six promised me that he liked her and that he was having fun. But I did tell her to stop pushing him to side-breathe. So, after two weeks of lessons, Six has learned a lot, but he hasn't learned to side-breathe. I don't worry about it. *He is six*, I think. *What does it matter?*

On the first day of swim practice—which is not, it is important to note, the Olympic qualifiers—Six has trouble remembering the coaches' instructions. Which stroke? Which lane? Swim
both ways or get out and walk around? There are lots of kids in
our tiny neighborhood pool, too many to count. Thirty? Forty?
It is hard for Six to tell which group he belongs with. Plus, there
are a dozen coaches, all screaming at different kids to do different things. Swim practice is, objectively, chaotic.

I realize that there is no way I could have previewed this. But
I decide not to worry. Sometimes it takes Six a couple of days
to get the feel for new things. We are members of this close-knit
pool club, and we paid to be on this swim team. I am certain
that they will give him a chance to get it right.

At home, I sometimes have to coach Six through basic tasks,
like getting dressed in the morning or brushing his teeth. Then,
other times, he does his tasks the first time I ask. When he forgets, he does what we call "doodling," when we get off track and
distracted by things. For example, I doodle when I start an email
five minutes before a videoconference with a client and then
look up and realize I'm five minutes late.

But always, no matter what, Six means well. When I find him
doodling and point it out, he jumps back to what he is supposed
to be doing, aware that he has made a mistake. He is aware, just
like I am.

While the coaches bellow at the children splashing in the
water, I sit on one of the lounge chairs, sunglasses on, acting
disinterested, but not at all disinterested. I cannot take Six,
or his brother, Eight, to any new place without paying close
attention to the care adults take with them. I have been too
well trained by how cruelly adults can treat kids, and kids like
mine in particular. It turns out I'm not wrong to be mistrustful
today.

Quick as a whip, Six is standing on the pool deck, and a coach, another white woman in her early twenties, is facing him. "You're supposed to be in that lane!" she yells, pointing at the pool where other six-year-old kids flop around like puppies.

"I'm sorry," Six says, voice audible to me over the screaming of coaches and the splashing and hollering of children.

The coach is befuddled by his ready apology. Like so many other adults in Six's life, she seems to believe that his mistake was intentional. "What is wrong with you?" she yells, a cruel question that adults fling around too often. The question is rhetorical. It actually means, *Something is wrong with you, and therefore you are bad.*

My son bursts into tears, saying, "I forget things."

The coach is taken aback by his direct and vulnerable answer. But she stays silent, offering no words of comfort in the face of his tears. Instead, she leads him back to his lane, and he hops in. After I make sure that he is safely back with his group, I stand from my chair, walk to the black metal fence hemming in the pool, grip two of the square metal posts, and weep behind my sunglasses.

Looking back, I should have pulled Six from the pool at that moment. At the very least, I should have talked with the coach and her supervisor about how her language is belittling in order to set her on a better path. Or I should have followed the doctor's advice to my mother thirty-five years ago and found someplace different or better, where social norms didn't crush and humiliate my child. But I didn't. I wanted my kid to have the joy of being on the neighborhood summer swim team. Excepting the moment on the pool deck, he was so happy to be there. He wanted to be with his big brother. He wanted to make the coach happy. So I let him stay and finish practice.

EXECUTIVE FUNCTION
AND WORKING MEMORY

Executive function (EF), as psychologists define it, is "a multi-dimensional cognitive construct that describes goal-directed, future-oriented behaviors."[6] In other words, EF is the part of your cognition, your very *thinking*, that governs anything you want to do in the future, even if that future is only one minute from now. These behaviors include planning, organizing, and even starting tasks; remembering things, like where you put your glasses or to brush your teeth; and controlling impulsivity.[7] Neurodivergent people, including kids with autism, ADHD, anxiety, and depression, tend to struggle with EF, as do kids who have experienced trauma.

My definition of executive function is slightly different from what you may find in the literature. As I define it, EF is the mental ability that people *use* to plan, concentrate, organize, exercise self-control, and manage daily tasks. I replace the typical "need" with "use" because "need" implies an inability to do those tasks if you struggle with EF. But I, like other neurodivergent people, *am* able to do complex tasks and remember things when I have the proper tools to assist me. For example, with alarms on my phone and a good calendar system, I can stay organized and manage time well. With a spreadsheet, I can plan a large project (like writing a book). I had to learn to use these tools, but I did learn. With these tools, I have strengthened my EF abilities, creating work-arounds that assist my struggles and capitalizing on my strengths (such as my technology skills).

Part of EF is "working memory." Working memory, according to psychologists, is "the process by which information is stored and processed mentally."[8] Working memory is like an inbox in our brains where information is put temporarily before either being permanently stored in a filing cabinet—our deeper memory—or discarded. For people with working memory struggles, that inbox doesn't work well or is missing completely. When information enters our working memory, the information just falls out again. In order for people who struggle with working memory to remember something, we must compensate, typically by bypassing working memory (the useless inbox) altogether and going straight to our deeper memory (the filing cabinet).

One strategy is to connect new information with information already in our deeper memory. For example, remembering names can be impossible for someone who struggles with working memory. After a person introduces themselves, the name is just gone—poof. So, when learning the name of a new person, we might associate something about the person with another person of the same name whom we already know. If I meet a person named Anne, for example, I try to find a characteristic about them that resembles my grandmother, who was also named Anne. I loved this grandmother very much, so when I think about her, I feel strong emotions, which generate strong memories.[9] If I meet a person named Anne who is tall like my grandmother was, I think, *Anne is tall like my grandmother Anne.* If she has thick, dark hair like my grandmother did, I think, *Anne has thick, dark hair like my grandmother Anne.* As I speak these words in my mind, I picture my grandmother standing next to the new Anne. If I do this memory work, I will rarely forget a name. In fact, I may never forget it because the name is now stored in my deep memory.

But doing this work at, say, a party with lots of new people is hard because the work-around takes time. I'm a neurodiversity advocate, so I don't mind asking for an extra moment to learn each person's name. I might say something like "Learning your names is important to me; let's take this slowly." The point is, these compensation tactics must be learned and practiced, often through trial and error, and they tend to be personal to an individual. This is not to say that I've overcome my struggle with names—hardly. I forget most names that I learn because I don't have the time or energy to do the work I just described. But the point is, I can if I need to.

When I was tested for autism in 2020, the scores on most of my cognitive abilities were high. My scores for EF, including working memory, were remarkably low by comparison. Comparatively low working memory is not unusual for some neurodivergent people. It doesn't reflect our intelligence, but it can seem to. For example, we can't cram for tests and score highly on them. We must actually learn the material, which takes longer. That means our test scores might be low in our AP exam–obsessed school culture, where deep learning is not the priority.

Before I was diagnosed with autism, I would get frustrated with myself, sometimes to the point of tears, wondering what was wrong with me that I couldn't remember the most basic things. I would lose my cell phone. I would send out emails with terrible typos. I would forget names and make people feel like they weren't important to me, even though they were. I would call myself stupid and careless—and things worse than that. After I saw my autism test scores and the doctor explained them to me, I learned how to give myself grace and to stop feeling humiliated and belittling myself. The thing is, I have never had trouble giving grace to my kids.

My kid, at six years old, talked with his private swim coach about electromagnetic pulses with deep expertise, but he struggled to remember which lane he was supposed to be in at swim practice. You can see how he might confuse adults who did not know him well. They might believe he was getting into the wrong lane on purpose. When the coach yanked him from the pool on the first day of swim practice and asked, "What is wrong with you?," she might as well have been asking, *How could such an intelligent child make such a stupid mistake?*

In response, Six told her his painful truth: "I forget things."

Put so simply, I wonder how anyone could fail to understand his struggle. But too many people do not understand, or do not want to understand, that people come in a glorious variety. And our society does not make space for variety. For some people and groups, the path for acceptable behavior is so narrow that it excludes even the most benign errors.

The psychiatrist my mom visited back when I was a child understood benign errors. She knew that trying to squeeze your kid into narrow acceptable norms was pointless and even harmful. She told my mother to trash those narrow norms and find better ones: *Find better people to carpool with.* Norms are not absolute. They're man-made and as change-able as the tides.

When you put ND people like me and my kids in chaotic en-vironments, keeping track of details is like navigating a tiny boat in a hurricane. The difference between children and adults is that adults have a greater ability to create work-arounds because of our maturity, life experiences, and resources. We also have a greater ability to stand up for ourselves, insisting that we be given what we need: time to process, a quiet space, a brain break, respect, and forgiveness. For many adults, however, ask-ing for these things can be hard because of the stigma attached to neurodivergence.

But a child must depend on the grace of adults, adults like a gentle and understanding swim coach who might give a kid some leeway, who might say, "It's okay that you forgot; just hop in this lane instead. I'm so glad you're here."

THE NARROW-MINDEDNESS OF ABLEISM

Two days later, on the third day of swim practice, Six seems to have the routine down. It has taken two days of navigating the chaos, but now he knows how to jump directly into the proper lane. He does everything the coaches ask. He guppies around with the other six-year-old kids, swimming as terribly and adorably as they do, back and forth, back and forth. He jumps out, joyfully, eager to do it again, and I am so happy for him.

I send a text message to my husband: **He's done it! Perfect swim practice!**

My husband texts back: **Yay buddy!**

I think about what we'll do at home to celebrate his outstanding swim practice. Toaster waffles with whipped cream? Homemade ice cream?

As I stand in the shade of a pool umbrella, admiring how well Six has adjusted to the chaos of swim practice, one of the coaches comes over to me. Let's call this coach Regina George. Regina is the same coach I hired to give Six private swim lessons for two weeks before the start of swim team. I hired Regina so that she could get to know Six. I figured if she spent time with him one-on-one, she would become accustomed to his quirks. She would see his gorgeous spirit in addition to his challenges. I was wrong about that. Never underestimate a person's desire to make her own life easier at the expense of a neurodivergent person.

Fifteen minutes before the end of swim practice, Regina tells me that Six is no longer welcome on the swim team.

I'm stunned and distraught, but I hide my feelings. "Why?" I ask calmly.

She doesn't answer my question. "We all met and decided together," Regina says, gesturing behind her at the entire coaching staff, the ten-plus high school and college-aged kids hollering on the pool deck, and the adult man who is their boss.

At her words, I imagine all of the coaches having a secret meeting to discuss the unworthiness of my child, and I want to scream.

"He requires too much individual attention," she says. "It isn't fair to the other kids."

Arguments leap to my mind to rebut her words, but I don't make them. I don't tell her about his perfect swim practice that day. I don't tell her that he just needed two days to adjust to a new chaotic environment and then will be fine going forward.

I certainly don't tell her that she could just give him less attention. They could stop focusing on whether he swims freestyle or backstroke so long as he's swimming laps, following safety instructions, and being kind and respectful to everyone at swim practice—which I know he is doing because I've been paying very, very close attention. Instead, I listen to her recount my child's failings, and I tell myself that I will not cry in front of a twenty-something swim coach.

Then she tells me that, in order to be on the team, Six needs to perform a list of tasks that I've never heard of before.

I shake my head at this. In the end, I'm autistic, which means I know the rules and can't abide dishonesty. Perhaps that's why I'm also a lawyer. "The prerequisites are listed on the website," I say. "It says that, to be on the team, a child needs to be able to swim one lap of the pool unassisted."

But Regina doesn't care that she changed the rules to exclude my child ex post facto. *After the fact.* At my words, she shrugs, and that is that.

I brush by her without a word—she's dead to me now—and then put a huge smile on my face as I extract Six and Eight from swim practice. I don't tell them why we're leaving early. They don't care. On the drive home, they chatter with each other in the back seat, always the best of friends.

As I drive, thoughts churn through my head. What do the coaches see when they look at my child? Why couldn't they give him one more day to get it right? Have they never before encountered a child who isn't the same as everybody else?

In my research for this book, one of the parent-interviewees, "Sophia," shared her perspective on the issue of kids fitting in: "When it comes to the social policing of neurodivergent people, they're pressured to conform to the least offensive, most bland version of acceptable behavior. Which really just sounds like society wants them to be not seen and not heard in public spaces."[10]

Recalling how I paid Regina hundreds of dollars to teach my child, I wonder, *Why is she now suddenly surprised by who he is?* Worse—Did my plan backfire? Did the lessons make Six a target? During those lessons, I told Regina that our goal was to help Six become accustomed to swim team and to give him the basic skills to succeed. I gave her details about things he struggles with, and she assured me she would be happy to work with him. But those lessons did, indeed, flag him as different from the other kids. Once the team practices started, he was no longer just another goofy six-year-old. He was the one Regina thought of as the kid who needs special attention because *I told her that he did.*

One thing I did not do was share a diagnosis with her. At the time, my gut told me it was wrong, and now, years later, my research confirms my gut feeling. Our children deserve their medical privacy. Revealing his medical diagnosis to one of an endless number of teenagers would only have harmed him. This was our neighborhood pool, an extension of our home. Six would grow up here. I'm grateful that I did not spill his diagnosis to the pool gossip mill. Plus, my son was not all that different from the other little kids on the team, so I had the privilege to keep his diagnosis secret.

So the big question is this: If Six had been just another kid in the crowd, would the coaches have seen his perfect swim practice that third morning and let him stay? In other words, would the coaches have cut him slack if he had been, to them, just another neurotypical face in the crowd?

As I drive home with the kids chattering in the back of the car, I think that today, at eight o'clock in the morning, when the water was freezing, and my Six climbed up on the starting block like a superhero with skinny arms, so brave, and jumped into the water and did the very best that he could—which is, if one is paying attention, *better* than the best that most six-year-old kids can do because most six-year-old kids aren't at a pool at eight o'clock in the morning—*that* is when they kicked him off of the team? He can never know about this small cruelty, I decide.

Is it small, though? Our swim team is society in microcosm. The narrow social norms at community swim don't stay at community swim, and they certainly weren't born there. These narrow norms are in schools, colleges, and workplaces. Neurodivergent people like me, Eight, and Six lose all sorts of opportunities because of the narrow-mindedness that our society's ableism encourages.

THE INDIVIDUAL ATTENTION FALLACY

If you're a parent reading this story, you might agree with Coach Regina George. You might be thinking, *Kids like yours take attention away from* my *kid.* But when the swim team coaches got together and decided that Six needed to go, they did not make that decision for Six's benefit or even the benefit of other children; they made it for their own. One less kid to pay attention to meant less work for them, especially when they made their jobs difficult by having a narrow concept of what correct behavior looked like.

"Individual attention" is frequently used as an excuse by neurotypical institutions to exclude ND kids (and adults) from camps, schools, teams, and clubs. But it is a fallacy that hides the real reason for exclusion. The "individual attention fallacy," as I call it, starts as a complaint from a group leader, such as a teacher or coach, that a ND person, usually a kid, is using more than their fair share of attention and therefore depriving it from neurotypical kids. But this complaint hides the reality that these leaders *choose* to spend their attention enforcing *irrelevant* norms, draining attention from everyone.

For example, the individual attention fallacy hides the fact that the swim coaches could spend less time enforcing irrelevant norms and rules such as "must swim backstroke and not freestyle in the six-year-old lane" instead of a more age-appropriate rule, such as "try backstroke, but if backstroke is too hard, just keep swimming and follow safety instructions." If they set aside irrelevant norms, leaders would have far more attention at their disposal. Attention is, indeed, zero sum, where giving attention to one person means that another must lose it. But it isn't ND kids who are draining the attention of leaders. It is what the leaders choose to spend their attention on.

In schools, for example, must students sit quietly and do nothing when they finish an assignment early, or is it okay for them to read a fun book or draw? Can they do so while sitting quietly on the floor instead of at their desks? Must students stand silently in straight lines waiting for lunch to start, or is it okay for them to talk to each other? Must students sit still in their seats and not wiggle, or is some fidgeting okay? Must students leave stuffed animals at home instead of holding them during class for comfort? If we start questioning all the norms that we take for granted, we can see how ND kids might not need much special attention at all. What makes so many of us different are the norms, not our neurodivergences.

Consider class discussions, from elementary school through high school and even college. Must students wait to be called on during class discussion, or is it okay to share their ideas when they pop in their heads—at least sometimes? And what about other ND kids whose processing speed is a little slower and they never get to speak because they take too long to raise their hands? Must they get punished for failing to participate? Teachers can develop other ways for them to participate, such as having everyone take a moment to write down their ideas first and then starting class discussion.

Freedom of movement, spontaneity, outlets for creativity: I'm describing a school environment where all children are allowed to be children, where ND kids, in particular, are allowed to be in their bodies (to "stim"), explore their special interests (e.g., by drawing trains, horses, or Minecraft maps when they have free time), and have other healthy outlets for their neurodivergences. Instead of squashing their neurodivergences to meet irrelevant norms of what a classroom is supposed to look like, ND kids are allowed to blossom like any other kid.

Rigid conformity to social norms is a cultural inheritance. Teachers and coaches are taught that the right way to do their job is to enforce conformity and allow no leeway. There must be straight lines, silence, compliance in all things. Otherwise, chaos reigns, right? (Wrong.) This rigidity can also be a manifestation of a lack of confidence. In my years of teaching, I've seen many insecure teachers trying to assert rigid control in the classroom because the students make them nervous. Norms make them feel safe. This lack of confidence makes teachers punish any transgression of irrelevant classroom norms. Confidence—via training, experience, or both—allows a teacher to tell the difference between what deserves their attention and what does not.

Despite my kids' gifts and because of their differences, it was a rare teacher who wanted one of my kids in their classrooms, and it was always apparent when they didn't. I received so many notes and emails recounting their screwups that eventually I put my husband's name on the school's contact list. I couldn't take any more of the emotional trauma required to read about my kids' supposed failures.

And yet, it is also true that some neurodivergent people *do* need more individual attention than others do; they have what are called greater "support needs."[11] Some neurodivergent people have higher support needs, and some (like me and my kids) have lower support needs. The reality of support needs is actually messier than that. Most of us have higher needs in certain areas and lower needs in others. The "spectrum" metaphor for autism (and other neurodivergences) never did represent our needs very well, and it is gradually being replaced with a "wheel," which resembles an artist's color wheel and allows for a person to identify their ND strengths and weaknesses across a variety of fronts, from executive functioning to emotional regulation to sensory challenges.[12]

A neurodivergent person with high support needs, who does indeed need more individual attention, also deserves a chance to participate in activities that fulfill them and bring them joy. So I return to a statement I made earlier: Is attention *really* a zero-sum game? Are there only a certain number of slices of the attention pie to go around? The answer, when viewed from another perspective, is no. If children with higher support needs wanted to join the swim team, the team could hire more coaches. They could make a bigger pie.

But enlarging the amount of attention to go around isn't always easy. Many, if not most, of our schools, after-school programs, and camps are understaffed and underfunded. This problem is structural, a problem that our society creates when our federal, state, and local governments make decisions about how to allocate our tax dollars, removing them from places that serve the public good like libraries, schools, and camps that take public funding.

Another structural problem is caused by ableism, where a program, such as a swim team, does not want to allocate funds for more coaches in order to be more inclusive. They'd rather do what our local pool did to me: kick the kid off the swim team and make me pay for private lessons instead. They shift the financial burden to the neurodivergent family, which is likely already overburdened, and not just financially. One of my parent-interviewees, Cameron, a Black woman and a parent of autistic children who has lived in both the South and in New York, laid it out plainly when talking about the camps her children attended.[13] She elected to send her kids to a publicly funded camp so that they could be around other Black children. But the camp was so poorly run it caused harm to her children. Cameron points out that treating "everybody the same" is not what inclusion of neurodiversity looks like. It is just a cost-cutting measure. When designing the camp for disabled and neurodivergent kids that her own kids attended, she explained, they didn't do anything unique for the kids in their care. Instead, she tells me, "They basically took a model for camps within the [town's] Parks and Recreation, including discipline [of children], and they lifted and shifted that model to the special needs camp." Furthermore, she told me that all of the camps were over capacity. In the end, she said, "You can't push everybody together to save money and call it inclusion because everybody loses. The typical children and the nontypical children lose. And the only people that gain are those people, the bureaucrats at the top who are getting six figures for nothing."

These structural problems pit teachers, school administrators, coaches, and camp counselors against parents and neurodivergent kids themselves. The kids aren't getting what they need (as I know from experience as both a kid and a parent), while teachers and so forth are overworked and underpaid. Everyone in the gladiator pit loses. But the fault doesn't lie with those of us in the pit fighting for scraps, rather with those in power who put us there, just as Cameron described.

The deciding factor in Six's case had to do with what the swim coaches chose to give their attention to. The coaches chose to pay attention to the ding-dong behavior of a gaggle of six-year-olds and tried to make the behavior stop. By choosing to enforce a narrow set of age-inappropriate behaviors, the coaches created a false crisis, activating the fallacy of individual attention. And then, when one particular six-year-old—my son—was more difficult to control than the rest, they culled him in order to make their lives easier.

Instead, they could have chosen to ignore everything other than the central task of summer swim team for the littlest children: to have the six-year-olds be safe, happy, and swimming. If the coaches had done so, they would have had attention left over for other kids who were struggling or sad—and even for ND kids with high support needs.

FIND THE RIGHT PLACES FOR YOUR KIDS

When my kids were first diagnosed with their neurodivergences, an endless list of long words and initialisms, I immediately called my mom. She told me about the wonderful child psychiatrist who'd helped her, and she reminded me about the carpool story, which I'd forgotten over the years.

She described her first meeting with the doctor, when she made this request: "I just want her to be like the other kids on the playground."

"She's never going to be like the other kids on the playground," the doctor said, shaking her head with a smile.

"But all of the other moms are going to think that my kid is a bad kid and that I'm a bad mom," my mom said.

"That's right," said the doctor. "That's exactly what they're going to think. And there's nothing you can do about it."

My mom told me that story the day I realized my own kids were never going to be like the other kids on the playground. I realized I'd been spending so many years avoiding the busy playground hours because the stress was too high. I couldn't bear to see the pinched faces of the other parents as they looked at my kids and thought terrible thoughts.

My kids have been kicked out of summer camp. Fired by piano teachers. Disallowed from group sports and relegated to private lessons instead. Threatened with expulsion from chess club. Back when I still tried to squeeze my kids into ableist groups, I lived in constant fear that I would receive a phone call telling me that yet another teacher, coach, or instructor decided to abandon them because they were too wiggly, chatty, distracted, or stubborn.

That's not to say that we haven't had incredible teachers, coaches, and instructors. We have.

My sons love playing piano and played in recitals since before their feet could touch the floor. But their first piano teacher
moved away. The second one died tragically young. So I hired a
third piano teacher from the same piano school, but she quit
after only three lessons, saying that my sons "aren't interested
in piano." After I got over my initial feelings of pain, I recognized
her words for what they were.

Bullshit.

I called the director of the piano school where my kids had
been students for years. But the director told me that I should
send my kids to choir instead of piano because my kids weren't
disciplined enough for piano. I asked for referrals to other piano teachers. She said she didn't have any. Suddenly it felt like
I was talking to a stranger, not the woman who had hugged my
children at recitals every fall and spring since they were small.

I started piano lessons very young. I was wiggly, defiant, distractible, and chatty. My piano teacher, who founded a preemi-
nent music school and later became far too famous to have ever
taught a mediocre musician like me, let me stand up during lessons. She let me talk while I played. She let me switch between
songs. She didn't care about any of those things because she
knew how to cultivate talent and joy. That was her job, and
she was very, very good at it. And because I wanted to make
her happy and she made me feel that joy, I practiced and practiced and practiced. I became far better at piano than I ever
should have. She wasn't a "special needs" piano teacher. She
was just a good one.

When I was a child, how many things, how many other
groups, how many teams was I thrown out of that my parents
never told me about? As an adult, I learned that my first-grade
teacher once told my parents that she wanted me out of her
class because I was too much for her to handle. Actually, she

called me "emotionally disturbed," words I find funny now, but that still hurt my mom a lot.

Curiously, in second grade, I was my teacher's favorite student. Until the day she died, she would send me cards on my birthday and hug me if we ran into one another in the grocery store. Her name was Mrs. Roberts. Mrs. Roberts never made me feel like I was made wrong. On the contrary—she made me feel like I was perfect. I still remember how she made me feel, even now, a lifetime later.

So the answer for us as parents of neurodivergent children is this: We must find better people to carpool with. We must surround our kids with Mrs. Robertses. This task is difficult, but it can be done.

One of my parent-interviewees, Anastasia, a white woman from New England, told me about discovering a place of acceptance for her trans-autistic kid (who uses the pronouns they/them) when she and her kid walked in a Pride parade together. She described the moment as "one of the most empowering things I've ever done, because I can say it was one of the first times that we've been together when I have seen them absorb acceptance, like physically feel accepted." At one point, her child "closed their eyes and just kind of took in the power of the support being showered upon everybody that was walking in the parade. And it was so moving. It was incredible." Finding a place where your child is accepted unconditionally can be hard, but it is possible. You just have to keep trying.[14]

Whenever I received emails and phone calls telling me that my kids were being thrown out of yet another activity, my first feeling was always grief for my kids. After all, I want them to have the chance to learn about the world and try amazing things. And as each door shut, those chances seemed to slip away. You might feel the same way. In those moments, reach for the three questions the child psychiatrist gave my mother: Did my kid put himself in danger? Did he put the other kids in danger? Did he damage property?

It isn't fair to throw a six-year-old off the swim team because he swam freestyle instead of backstroke. After all, he didn't put himself in danger, or other kids, or property. I know those things were true because I watched, and I asked. Regina and her fellow coaches simply thought Six was annoying.

But what if a kid is disruptive in a classroom or a sports team to the point that the coach cannot coach or the teacher cannot teach? It is true these things happen. Sometimes the issue is that a student has higher support needs than the teacher or coach is prepared to supply, and they need more resources. As the individual attention fallacy shows, if the kid does need more attention than the resources allow, it isn't the kid's fault. The fault lies with the system that withholds those resources.

If a child who doesn't appear to have higher support needs "acts out," the question we must answer is what happened ten minutes before. Kids don't do things for no reason. Did your kid start stimming? Did your kid run from the classroom? Ask yourself this: Why would *you* shake or flap in distress or run from a classroom? Why would anyone? The answer is simple: Something made that child feel unsafe, and we need to figure out what it was.

My children have had teachers who made them feel safe every day. They have also had teachers who caused harm, when after school they came home in shaking distress and slept for two hours. Based on experience and research, I know it is possible to do it right. We just have to care enough, as a society, to include neurodivergent kids inside the group of "normal."

When Coach Regina George recited the litany of fake reasons that they needed Six off the team, she didn't realize she needn't have bothered to lie. I would never leave my kid in a place where he's not wanted. If we have the choice, we must never leave our children in a place where they are not wanted. They will be neglected at best and abused at worst, even if the abuse doesn't show as bruises on the body. The psychological damage, according to child abuse experts, is just as harmful. It hurts to be told that you're made wrong, that you're too loud, too weird, too *much*. The damage I suffered at the hands of those who had power over me has never eased, even after decades.

The question is simple: Is there room for neurodivergent kids at a piano school? On a swim team? In most classrooms? The answer, right now, seems to be no. Instead, as parents, it is our job to surround our children with love, affirmation, and acceptance.

The day Six was kicked off of the swim team, we got home from the pool, and I sent the kids upstairs to get dressed. Then I called my mom. I asked her to tell me the old story about the preschool carpool. She told me that she was at a cocktail party when the Mean Girls of the carpool informed her that I was no longer welcome in their station wagons. "One of the fancy moms told me how much you'd misbehaved in her car," my mom said. (She actually used the phrase "fancy moms.") "So the next day, I went to preschool early to pick you up before the regular carpool mom could arrive because I couldn't bear to see her."

My mom sat in the room at preschool where parents could watch the kids through the one-way mirror. The room was kept dark to make it easier to see the kids. In that small, dark room, she cried, watching me, knowing the bad things that the fancy moms had said about me in secret, carrying that knowledge while I played in the room, innocent and unknowing.

When she told me this story, I knew exactly what she'd felt. It's how I felt when Regina told me about the secret swim coaches' meeting. While Regina spoke to me that morning, I didn't look at her. Instead, I looked over her shoulder, watching Six jump off the diving block, freezing at 8:00 A.M. practice, doing the very best he could. While he worked hard with an enormous grin on his face, I already knew he couldn't come back the next day. While Regina was listing his faults, he was doing everything he could to make the coaches happy, not knowing that it would never be enough.

My mom asked me, "What are you going to tell him?"

"What did you tell me?"

"I didn't tell you until you were in high school. By then, you thought it was funny."

Six is now Thirteen, and his brother is Fifteen, and I still haven't told them about the awful day at swim team or all of the other days when they were rejected from places that should have welcomed them. One day, when we're all older and firmly self-assured, we will laugh, together.

As families, we must fight for classrooms where neurodiversity is affirmed, not punished. Find extracurricular spaces where our kids are showered in love. Do not allow one moment of harm to go unanswered. You are not asking for too much, I promise. You don't have to wait for the benefit of hindsight. Use mine.

And if you're reading this after already making the mistakes I did, I promise it isn't too late. Every time your child sees you stand up for them, they will trust you more. Every time that you listen to them tell you a story about harm they suffered at the hands of a bully—whether a child or an adult—and you believe them wholeheartedly, they will trust you. That trust is the foundation of the relationship with your child. If you listen, and you believe, then they will come to you with their secrets. Then together you can build a world where they can thrive.

CHAPTER 2

Previewing, Meltdowns, and Social Policing

When I was a kid, I hated Christmas.

At the time, I didn't realize that I did. Like every other kid, I got excited when the weather turned cold, when Christmas carols came on the radio, when it was time to have my picture taken with Santa, and when I decorated the tree with my parents. But some things about Christmas are hard for neurodivergent people. At Christmastime, there's a lot of chaos and unpredictability. Schedules change. It's hard to keep track of days, of time. Of anything. And then there's the forced happiness: Everyone is expected to be joyous. If we are lucky enough to have received presents, we are supposed to be delighted for them even if they're terrible. At the holidays, ND kids are expected to be so happy, all the time.

As kids, the purpose of our holiday happiness is, in part, to make the adults happy. Even a socially awkward kid like me could figure that out. After getting it wrong a few times when I opened my gifts—the excitement building, the box opening, the gift disappointing, my face falling—my mother took me aside and taught me the script: "Thank you for the present. It's perfect." Or, "Thank you for the present. I will use it all the time." These words, delivered with a false smile, were meant to keep adults happy.

But the pressure to please the adults around me was a lot. There were the adults giving the gifts, such as my innumerable aunts, uncles, and older cousins. And then my parents, on whom, it seemed, my every misstep reflected poorly. Because of that pressure, because of that chaos, I cried every single Christmas from the time I was old enough to know what Christmas was. Indeed, I still cry at Christmas sometimes.

You might think that my parents, when confronted by their child weeping under the Christmas tree, would ask, "What's wrong?" You might expect that they would try to comfort me. But my parents were so stunned, so flabbergasted, by my Christmas tears, and my reaction so opposite of what they expected, that they usually responded with aggravation or anger. "Why are you crying?" my mother would ask, an edge to her voice.

"I don't know," ten-year-old me would reply, heaving with sobs.

"How can you not know?"

My brain was swirling, my stomach filled with knife-wing butterflies. I felt awful, and I couldn't say why. And so my parents sighed, and they walked away.

I understand their pain. I must've been a shock. If you're a parent, then you know how it goes: You stay up all night on Christmas Eve, assembling toys and wrapping presents. What if *your* kid cried all over the gifts? From the outside, I must have seemed like a brat, throwing a tantrum because I didn't get the gifts I wanted. But that wasn't the problem at all. It was the chaos and surprises of the holidays. At the time, I wasn't able to articulate the reason for my tears. And that inability to explain made everything worse.

But we know, today, that these ND expressions of emotions need not be bad. They are a healthy release of pent-up anxiety and fear. At those times when we can't shelter our kids from needless chaos, we can create a space where they can be safe cleansing themselves of negative feelings.

THE ANIMAL SHELTER

It's my son Nine's birthday. We're heading to the animal shelter after school to adopt a cat for his gift. He's been planning this outing for weeks. We let him know a long time ago what his gift would be. We set the parameters for what kind of cat we could get: He must be male and under the age of four, to ease the relationship with the older female cat we already have, but not a kitten. Nine knew just what he wanted: a Maine Coon cat, the largest domesticated cat in the world, according to his research.

"Baby," I say. "They're not going to have a Maine Coon cat at the shelter."

Because my kid is neurodivergent, I need to work a little harder to help him manage his expectations—that is, to preview what is to come. If we don't talk about things in advance, he will feel crushing disappointment when there is no Maine Coon cat, and his emotions might overwhelm him. His expression of his disappointment might be tears or even a meltdown. These are ND behaviors that bystanders, even members of his own extended family, would perceive as overblown, childish, or spoiled.

Although he's been to the shelter before and it seems like there is a vast number of cats, it can be hard for a kid to understand that there is only a limited selection. Any kid, neurotypical or neurodivergent, might feel that way. Therefore, any kid can benefit from having an adult with greater experience smooth the way.

After pondering my words about the unlikelihood of finding the exact cat he's dreaming of, he says, "That's okay. We'll find a good one."

With enough notice, my kid—like any kid—can go along with anything.

On the day we planned, my husband and I come home early from work. As a family, we head to the shelter, a thirty-minute drive from our house. We arrive an hour and a half before they close. We have plenty of time to visit with the animals, select our pet, fill out the paperwork, and bring the cat home. We've brought all the supplies they require, according to their website: a carrier, a towel, identification, and a checkbook.

When we enter the shelter and see the myriad cats in their small houses, I can tell Nine is overwhelmed by the choices. I'm glad that we set parameters of age and sex to narrow our search.

The first and only cat we find that meets our parameters is Miles, a black tuxedo, just like our other two cats at home. Miles instantly bonds with Nine in the visiting room. But my husband and I aren't sure. How could it be that there is only one cat at the shelter that meets our criteria? So I walk around the shelter once more, looking closely at each cat to make sure we do not miss another one of the right age and sex. Pulling aside a sign partly blocking the view, I find one cat we overlooked.

There, behind a pane of glass, sits a majestic Maine Coon mix, all golds and reds, a veritable feline giant, face pressed up against the glass in an inquiring expression.

I call out to Nine, "Come here!"

He comes running over, his sneakers slapping against the polished concrete floor.

"What do you see?" I say to him.

He reads the words on the sign carefully. Then, my kid does what every parent loves to see: He loses his complete shit with joy.

"Mom! You said they wouldn't have one!"

"I did, buddy." I smile, unable to stop. "I was wrong."

We take the miniature lion into the visiting room. Nine is very good with cats. He reads manuals and handbooks about them. He studies them on the internet. He is a cat expert. Like Miles did, the cat takes to him immediately, ignoring me, recognizing the gentle child who will be his friend. The cat, whom my kid has already named Goldeneye, is perfect.

Thirty minutes before the shelter closes, while my son hands the cat to the workers in the cat room to get the cat ready to go home, I head up to the counter to pay and sign the paperwork.

"Sorry," the lady at the desk tells me. "No adoptions thirty minutes before closing."

The breath whooshes from my body like I've taken a surprise tackle from behind. For a moment, I can't speak. I run through the details in my brain, all of the research I did before we came. I know this thirty-minute rule isn't on the website. I read the posted rules on the signs around the building. I know everything that the public could possibly know because I researched it, all of it, before we came. My heart is racing, but I lock my emotions down tight.

"Is there a way we were supposed to know that?" I ask. "We've been here for an hour, and we would have come up here sooner if we had known."

"It's the rule," she says. "Sorry."

She doesn't sound sorry. She sounds apathetic. She doesn't know what her words are doing—to me, right now, and what they will do to my son. I think of the time we spent as we dawdled in the playroom with Goldeneye. If only I had stepped out five minutes sooner. If only I hadn't stopped to chat with the volunteer in the cat room.

The woman at the counter is telling me, right now, that my child is going to be crushed in a very specific way. A way I would have been crushed when I was his age. A way that I'm being crushed right now—in echoes I've learned to ignore but that have never gone away.

Adaptability to sudden change can be difficult for neurodivergent minds. As psychologist Megan Anna Neff explains, "Sometimes, as neurodivergent people, we struggle to adapt to change, stress, and conflict. More often than neurotypicals, we experience panic attacks, anxiety and depression disorders, difficulty regulating our emotions, and more." The reason for these struggles has to do with the differences in the nervous systems of ND people: "When our nervous systems are rigid (have a small window of tolerance) because of neurodivergence or trauma, we can easily fall into dysregulation, characterized by hyperarousal and hypoarousal."[1] In other words, ND kids (and adults) have nervous systems that more easily dysregulate in moments of sudden change and conflict.

Neurotypical families might show up to adopt a pet and discover they needed a checkbook but didn't bring one. These families might feel strong disappointment and sadness. But "strong disappointment" does not describe the powerful emotional reactions of my neurodivergent family to the sudden loss of Goldeneye. Shrugging things off is not our strength. We don't feel disappointment, we feel like the world has tilted sideways and that it will never right itself again. So our family did everything we could to make things predictable. We followed the rules down to every detail. We accommodated the animal shelter. We would *never* expect them to accommodate us.

But now, at the metal counter, twenty-nine minutes before closing, I am asking for just that. "Is there anything we can do? We just want to adopt a cat. We've been here for an hour." I'm begging.

"No."

If I stepped up to the counter one solitary minute earlier, we would be bringing Goldeneye home. My failure feels catastrophic. I want to cover my face with my hands, fall to my knees, and let out the volcano of emotions that her words just created inside of me.

Instead, I suppress the churning in my gut, my shaking hands, and the rest of the strong emotions, just like I've done for most of my life. But I'm unable to suppress them completely because the feelings erupt as tears. Tears are more socially acceptable than sobbing and shaking on the floor, but they're still an odd reaction from a grown woman. To hide my tears, I turn quickly from the counter, reacting to the decades of shame that I've internalized. I don't want the worker to see my slip in control. For me to have a meltdown, even a small one, is disgraceful.

Worse, I know that Nine is going to be even more devastated than I am, and he will likely have a meltdown. If the lady at the counter sees him, Nine will look like he is having a tantrum. He will look like a spoiled brat who didn't get his way. But he isn't a brat. Nine is the opposite of spoiled.

To break the news to Nine, I take him around the corner from the entrance, behind some shrubs, and hold him while he lets out all of his feelings. I affirm for him how unfair it is and listen when he tells me how worried he is that Goldeneye will be gone tomorrow before I rush back to adopt him. He leans into me while he sobs. He feels like he might die because of this misshapen day. But I don't shame him for his pain. Holding him,

I tell him it's okay to feel his feelings. Then I tell him, fiercely, that I will make it right.

It has taken me years to have that kind of compassion for myself, and only after I received an autism diagnosis and lots of psychotherapy to aid in self-understanding and self-acceptance.

PREVIEWING

When my family reviewed all of the rules of the shelter to prepare for our visit and talked to Nine about the kind of cat he would likely find, we were "previewing." We previewed to make sure that our family knew what to expect at the shelter and during the adoption process. We were able to talk through scenarios at home so that we could feel all of our feelings there, in a safe place, before heading out into public. Previewing helps ND kids (and adults) keep their emotions regulated because it prevents the kinds of surprises that activate our nervous systems.

In occupational therapy research, previewing is defined as a "behavioral intervention which involves the previewing of an activity or materials in a low-demand, high-reinforcement context prior to performance."[2] To help ND kids prepare for a new activity, therapists, teachers, or parents perform the new activity in a safe place (one that is "low demand") where the kid feels comfortable in their surroundings, and hopefully the kid will therefore gain comfort with the activity, too. If the previewing works, when the time comes to do the activity in the "real" space, the activity is no longer new or uncomfortable.

But previewing should be more than a "behavioral intervention," or a focus on changing a kid's neurodivergent behavior traits to make them appear more neurotypical. Behavioral interventions put the focus on the comfort of the people *around* the neurodivergent kid. The problem is, whenever we force our kids to act more neurotypical, we cause them harm.[3] A neurodiversity-affirming ("neuroaffirming") approach does not view neurodivergence as something to be corrected but rather as a normal part of human diversity with struggles to be supported and strengths to be embraced.

Previewing, like other therapies for ND kids, can be neuroaffirming.[4] The goal of neuroaffirming previewing is not to make neurodivergent kids act neurotypical but to ensure that they can enjoy a new experience. Thus, in my research, I've come up with a definition of previewing that is neuroaffirming: It is when you let someone know what is coming so that they can manage their expectations properly and prepare for it both mentally and with tools if necessary—especially when, because of how their brains are wired, it is a little harder for them to handle the unexpected than it is for other people.

Previewing can greatly reduce a ND person's anxiety about a new person, place, or activity, and it can give them confidence. The two things are closely related. If you are anxious, it is hard to feel confident taking part in an unfamiliar activity.[5] For example, in one study, the day before an autistic child joined a group setting with autistic and neurotypical kids, a psychologist played a board game with the autistic child, keeping the game low stakes and fun and frequently telling the child that the game would be played the next day.[6]

But by my definition, the burden of previewing is not only on the neurodivergent kid but also on the neurotypical person or group who will be spending time with the neurodivergent kid. In other words, the ND kid doesn't have to carry the load of the new experience alone. Instead, the adults in charge of the new experience have a duty to help the kid find ways to feel safe and enjoy the new experience.

In an email interview about previewing, pediatric speech and language pathologist Jessie Mewshaw, a white woman who is an ADHDer and also a parent of two neurodivergent kids, explained to me that previewing can and should be more expansive than just ensuring that a kid is able to behave well in a new environment. Sure, she told me, "the unexpected is anxiety-provoking, and a preview allows some of the unknown to be more known."[7] But previewing, Mewshaw explained, is also about collaborating with the ND kid to create "proactive strategies and accommodations that could be relevant for the new thing." Mewshaw explained that the goal of this tactic "is empowering the client." For example, if the new place is going to be loud (such as a musical event on a school field trip), then a preview should include not only the information about what the trip will entail but also a collaboration with the kid about how to handle the noise, such as a plan to bring noise-canceling headphones to use when the kid gets overwhelmed.

One tool for previewing is a "social story." A social story is a story written by a counselor or someone similar, told from the child's point of view, often with illustrations, that includes "what the child might not understand and how they can successfully navigate the event or activity."[8] Sometimes social stories are not neuroaffirming, in which case they dictate behaviors the child should perform in order to mimic neurotypicals. But the better social stories help ND children navigate confusing environments and empower them to make good decisions on their own.

As an adult, I've learned over time how to preview for myself. It took me far longer than it should have to figure out that I needed to do this preparation. For example, when I have a work trip now, I study the details of my travel plans, look at possible interruptions and think about how I will handle them, start packing days in advance to ensure I have planned out my needs, and so on. By taking these measures, I create confidence that I can handle the potential chaos that traveling might throw my way. Even still, I sometimes break down when the chaos is too much, such as when I'm stuck in an airport while a kid is sick at home and I'm desperately trying to get there.

But kids can't do previewing work for themselves. We have to help them. When they're small, we must preview for them and collaborate on tools that might help them. As they get older, we must teach them the skills to understand not only that their needs are valid but also how to make sure their needs are met. We can teach our kids to feel empowered to ask for what they need.

MELTDOWNS AND SHUTDOWNS

But what happens when a neurodivergent kid—or adult—winds up in a situation that couldn't be adequately previewed? Where the planning falls apart and disaster strikes? Kids can be overcome by emotions that need to be let out, like steam from an overloaded valve. That's when a meltdown occurs. I define a neurodivergent meltdown as a strong emotional response to sensory or emotional overload, caused by either the buildup of small events or one large event, that releases the emotional overload and allows the person to regulate their emotions. Meltdowns can appear as sobbing, anger, or other strong emotions.[9]

Meltdowns happen when neurodivergent kids (and adults) become *dysregulated*, that is, unable to emotionally manage the stressors we encounter. When that happens, we lose our internal self-control. As Amanda Diekman, autistic author and neurodiversity parenting expert, explains, dysregulation means stress, and "kids who are stressed are not able to make the best choices." These poor choices look like bad behavior to adults, but, as Diekman points out, "This behavior is actually a stress response, not a behavioral one."[10] Diekman explains that a meltdown is a stress response brought on by dysregulation, a symptom of "acute anxiety overload, a panicked brain caught in the survival pathway, unable to find a way to return to steady calm."[11] Meltdowns happen not only to children. Teens, young adults, and women in their forties at animal shelters will melt down or shut down as well.[12]

Emmy-Award–winning neurodivergent comedian Hannah Gadsby writes about meltdowns and shutdowns in their memoir: "My meltdowns had always been a mystery to me, so when I was finally diagnosed [as an adult], I was able to reframe the way I thought about my strange little outbursts. For a start, I became far more compassionate toward myself, which probably halved the distress of the occasions."[13] Gadsby's words about self-compassion resonate with me as a late-diagnosed adult because that's the main thing I've had to learn. Then Gadsby describes the negative—and positive—aspects of meltdowns: "A meltdown is a maelstrom that begins in the body," but meltdowns can also be "a real spring clean. They clear the pipes and can often leave you feeling as if your body has been reset."[14]

But, Gadsby points out, they themselves haven't had many meltdowns because they are "more of a shutdown kind of autistic." Like meltdowns, shutdowns are also not socially acceptable: "From the outside, a shutdown looks very similar to a sulky tantrum." But, they explain, a shutdown isn't a tantrum because the person does not have control over themselves. Gadsby's metaphor for a shutdown is "like a maxed-out power grid in the middle of a storm."[15]

In my own experience and research, I've seen how shutdowns have a similar function to meltdowns. As autistic psychologist

Devon Price describes them, shutdowns are "essentially a way of dissociating from one's surroundings. It can look like falling asleep very suddenly, becoming unresponsive, or just kind of zoning out."[16] Price writes in the context of autism, but shutdowns can happen to other neurodivergent people, such as those who have experienced trauma or those with anxiety. Neurodivergent meltdowns or shutdowns, no matter how they manifest, are never acceptable under our society's social norms. And that's a whole different problem.

SOCIAL POLICING

Parents of neurodivergent kids know that shutdowns and meltdowns are not socially acceptable because people around us let us know. Sometimes, when our kid is melting down, a family member says something unintentionally (or intentionally) cruel. Sometimes a stranger in a store gives us a dirty look. The judgment of our parenting, and of our children, is painful. The only cure is a stout sense that what you are doing as a parent is right and what your child is expressing is normal and okay. But it can be hard to get there.

In her book *Autism in Heels*, autistic author and advocate Jennifer Cook O'Toole (a white woman) tells the story of a day when her daughter had a meltdown during school: "She was worn out, embarrassed, lonely, and miserable, and that day, she totally lost it—sobbing and screaming outside the classroom, unwilling to go in." Instead of having sympathy for O'Toole's kid, the teacher shamed O'Toole: "In a phone call later that evening, the teacher interrogated us. 'I am just wondering,' she asked curtly, 'if you ever discipline this child?' "[17] The teacher then expressed doubt that O'Toole's daughter even had a diagnosis of Asperger's (a subtype of autism). O'Toole pushed back against the teacher's mistreatment of her and her child, defending her and pointing out the teacher's ignorance of neurodiversity. But most autistic children do not have neurodiversity advocates for parents or parents who can easily withstand the compounded criticism of our children by family, teachers, coaches, camp counselors, and strangers at the grocery store.

Research supports that parents of ND kids face intense scrutiny and judgment when they take their kids out in public. This "social policing" by others is an attempt to force ND kids into conforming with rigid social norms. The research shows that, for *all* families, "surveillance" by other adults in public spaces socializes children (and their parents) into what is considered socially appropriate behavior.[18] These social rules don't serve a functional purpose, such as public safety. Instead, they are rules derived from ableist social norms meant to keep everyone "normal."[19]

Because of social policing, parents of ND kids learn quickly that "the streets belong to adults and children" who are not like them.[20] When they do go out in public, ND families are ostracized by other adults, sometimes with words but frequently with more subtle behavior. Other adults use "stares, glares or comments" to police the behavior of ND families.[21] These stares and glares are a silent yet painful enforcement of social norms. Parents whose children "create disorder" in public suffer because this disorder "directly reflects on the perceived competence" of the parents.[22] When ND kids violate social norms, their parents "often appear to be incompetent parents" rather than parents of kids who experience the world in a different, yet normal, way.[23] As an example, think back to the teacher who scornfully questioned O'Toole's parenting skills. For the teacher, the daughter's meltdown was evidence that O'Toole was a terrible mom.

When a neurodivergent kid melts down, shuts down, or otherwise breaks social norms in public, they become "social rule breakers" and are publicly shamed.[24] This public shaming of ND families causes parents to do immense emotional work to ensure that their families avoid breaking social rules. Yet, at the same time, research shows that parents are deeply protective of their children. They ensure that their children are shielded from the mean behavior of outsiders. Performing this double duty of minimizing public disruption while protecting their children comes at a great cost to the parents' emotional well-being.[25]

Parents in these studies noted that public interactions are the "hardest thing to deal with" of all of their parenting dilemmas. Their children, they reiterated, were not the problem. Other people were. This fact highlights the power of public encounters and shaming in our everyday lives.[26] Wonderfully, parents in these studies did not felt shame toward their children or their children's ND behaviors or identities. In fact, "parents demonstrated an empathetic understanding of their children's sensory sensitivities" and struggled not with their kids but with outsiders who tried to shame their families.[27] The researchers note, in the context of autism, that because of these painful public encounters, families tended to self-isolate to avoid them: "The combination the intense distress public places can create for children with ASD, the effect of the disciplinary gaze and lack of understanding often shown by people present and the emotional turbulence this creates for the parents, led parents to take their children out less," which causes emotional harm to ND families.[28]

Neurodivergent emotional expression must also be viewed intersectionally, taking into account gender, race, and more. We live in a society where norms insist that boys shouldn't cry, so when a ND boy cries, he violates two social norms. Norms insist that Black women avoid emotional expressions that might be perceived as the stereotypical "angry Black woman" outburst. Thus, for ND Black women, *any* emotional outburst puts them at risk of social ostracization. Even more tragically, Black men— and women as well—must avoid anything that appears aggressive; otherwise, they risk endangering themselves in encounters with police. For Black boys and men, emotional dysregulation in stressful situations can, quite literally, be deadly.[29]

Take the story of Olivia Brown, a Black autistic woman from Birmingham, England, who melted down in public in her early twenties after a stressful event—a trial in which her rapist was found not guilty. Outside after the trial, as Olivia recounted to autistic author and activist Kala Allen Omeiza, "Olivia 'erupted' into stims and wails made from overstimulation." Police were present at the courthouse, but rather than coming to the aid of a distressed woman, they "feared for themselves instead." As the police called for backup, Olivia's meltdown grew worse under the added stress they caused. Then, something special happened: "Finally, a Grenadian security guard pulled Olivia up and stroked her hair. The Black security guard pulled her close until her breathing slowed, and the cloud [of her meltdown] vanished."[30] But most police do not see ND people in distress, especially ND people of color, as in need of comfort but rather in need of restraint and punishment.

If institutions such as schools and workplaces are going to claim to be inclusive of neurodiversity, then they must also accept the various emotional expressions that are part of being neurodivergent. But there is a distinct lack of understanding of neurodivergent emotional expression. When a ND kid melts down after a disappointment, neurotypical social norms perceive the behavior to be "bad" because that is the only explanation under our current social norms for such an emotional expression. And, as Olivia's story shows, punishment of ND emotional expression only creates more stress that needs to be released, creating a miserable and sometimes dangerous (to the ND person) cycle.

As parents, the only solution is to gain greater confidence in our parenting and greater understanding of our ND kids—both so that we can avoid putting them in situations that cause them to dysregulate (which harms them) but also so that we can stand up to the social policing that we face every day.

HYPERVIGILANCE

Because of social policing, when we as parents spend any amount of time in public with our ND kids, we can become "hypervigilant" about how other people see our families. This hypervigilance is difficult to discard even when you find deep acceptance of yourself and your children because it becomes so ingrained.

While researching this book, I interviewed Sophia, the parent of a fourteen-year-old son who is autistic and has ADHD (AuDHD). Sophia is a straight, white, cisgender woman in a heterosexual marriage.[31] Sophia told me that the social policing of her and her child started when he was a toddler. Her son didn't communicate in words until around his third birthday. "Which meant," Sophia told me, "that every time I would take him out into public, like the grocery store," she faced social pressure from outsiders. She told me, "You can't push a cute kid around in the wagon without lots of old folks wanting to stop and make conversation." They would talk to her kid, "and my kid didn't answer." At the time, Sophia didn't know her son was neurodivergent, but she "got all these comments from people on my kid.

Lack of response, lack of engagement." She felt "this pressure to say something, to try and gloss over the fact that my kid wasn't answering people. It always felt like trying to smooth the ripples."

Sophia struggled with how to respond to these suspicious adults who felt free to share their observations about her kid: "You know, you've got a shy kid," they would say. "And meanwhile my kid is sitting there listening to this, and I'm like, I don't know if he's shy or not, really. But I don't want him to start taking on this label." She knew he wasn't verbal, but she also knew he could understand. What Sophia describes is the unwelcome social policing forced on her as a parent of a ND kid by outsiders who invited themselves into interactions with her and her son, causing her great distress because she was worried about both protecting him from pushy statements and, at the same time, lowering social tensions. Looking back on it now, she realized that she was in a constant state of protective hypervigilance whenever she entered a public space that was not designed for kids like hers.

One time, when Sophia was able to drop this hypervigilance in public, she realized how ingrained her hypervigilance had become. After her son received a diagnosis of neurodivergence at age five, she went to a gathering for other ND kids and families. She described to me a small moment of acceptance that was life-changing to her: "Inside the lunch tent, my son started throwing food and utensils, and I immediately felt very anxious." But instead of shaming Sophia, the other adults accepted her son's anxious outburst as normal: "Other parents walking by just plucked the things up from the ground and set them on the table and kept walking." To the other adults in the group, her son's behavior "was a nonevent. I realized that I nearly cried because I felt this pressure leave me." As she told me, she realized that, because of how the other adults acted, the gathering was "a safe space." The experience was eye-opening because it "made me realize how much tension I was usually carrying, that I had gotten so used to feeling. I wasn't always aware of it until that event, when I felt it lift." The hypervigilance that Sophia describes and the desire to smooth the ripples are pressures that many parents of ND kids can relate to. So what can we do to help us set aside these pressures?

Neurodivergent expressions of emotions often seem overblown to neurotypical outsiders, so the burden falls on ND people to keep our emotions in check. Many, if not most, ND adults and parents of ND kids work hard to protect neurotypical people from having to deal with our emotions, even if we don't realize we're doing it. We know that ND emotional expressions do not garner sympathy. Instead, they garner scorn, judgment, and sometimes violence. And, like most social norms, the narrow scope of acceptable emotional expression in our neurotypical world harms any person who might need to express emotions beyond the limited ones that our society permits, whether neurodivergent or neurotypical.

REJECTING SOCIAL POLICING OF OUR KIDS

The day my family leaves the animal shelter without Goldeneye, we don't go straight home. The kids, especially Nine, need a distraction from their sadness. So we go to a fast-food restaurant, an unusual treat, and let them order whatever they want. The distraction works for a little while—at least Nine's sobbing has stopped while he sadly eats his fries. But I am not distracted. My heart is still racing, and I feel like I have to do something. "Give me your laptop," I tell my husband, who always carries it with him. "They'll listen if the email is from a dad."

There, at the bright-yellow table in the fast-food restaurant, I draft a straightforward email to the shelter director, just the facts about what happened with the timing of our arrival, the staff, and the arbitrary and invisible cutoff time. I make sure there is no anger in the letter. I mention that Nine is neurodivergent and that his disappointment was strong after we followed all the rules. I sign off with my husband's name and send it because in our society, men—fathers—get more respect when they stand up for their kids; women/mothers are too emotional. (These stereotypes, and the binaries themselves, are nonsense, of course.) Ending the email, I make only the small request that they ensure the information on their website is accurate.

Minutes later, I receive a reply from the director of the animal shelter. As I read it, I'm shocked.

He apologizes, deeply and sincerely. He says that he wants to know the details of what happened and hopes to apologize to us in person. He tells me that Goldeneye will be ready for us to pick up first thing in the morning. And finally, he says that his own kid is neurodivergent and he gets it, he really does.

When I receive the email, an emotional overload hits me once again. All of the strength I have been using to hold up the world for my family gives out, and I crash, crying once more.

A few emails later, the director and I have arranged a phone call. I get up to speak to him outside, my tears under control again. Surrounded by the stench of oil from the deep fryer, I plan to meet him in the morning when the shelter opens. He apologizes again and tells me he looks forward to meeting me.

At bedtime that evening, as I tuck Nine into bed, I make a promise. "He'll be waiting for you when you get home from school."

Nine is thrilled, and he flops back onto his pillow with a smile on his face.

The morning after my stifled meltdown at the shelter, I arrive back there and park out front. Rather than feeling thrilled to pick up Goldeneye, I feel sick to my stomach. Memories from the day before come flooding back—the urgency I felt in my gut, the tears I shed. Decades of hiding my own autistic expression made me ashamed of expressing my feelings. Now I feel exhausted and hungover.

Taking a deep breath, I climb from the car, lugging the oversized cat carrier. At the counter, I'm deliberately calm, pitching my voice low, acutely aware of how I lost control while standing at this counter the day before and feeling embarrassed all over again. I feel like I used to feel when I was a child after a meltdown—because, in retrospect, I *had* a meltdown. I just didn't know it at the time because I was yet-to-be autistic and had no one to teach me about my own emotional expression. When Goldeneye couldn't come home with us, I masked my emotions. I now know that taking the churning in my gut, the tears, and the shaking and squeezing them down deep inside me is unhealthy. I sometimes make myself physically sick rather than feel the shame of letting my emotions free. Like most ND kids, I learned young how to mask my feelings in order to stay safe. As psychologist Devon Price explains, in the context of autistic kids, "When they're told their stigmatized traits are just signs that they're a disruptive, overly sensitive, or annoying kid, they have no choice but to develop a neurotypical façade."[32] That day at the shelter, my lifelong façade—my mask—slipped, and I felt deeply ashamed.

Weeks later, as I reflected on my family's meltdowns at the shelter, I called my mom to speak to her about how I used to cry at Christmas. She said, "We were terrible to you. You would cry, and your dad and I would get so upset with you." I told her that I don't blame her. My parents did the best they could with the tools they had. Being yelled at for crying on Christmas hurt me, yes. To have someone get angry at me when I melted down under the stress of the holidays reinforced the shame I felt surrounding meltdowns, and so I subconsciously suppressed those meltdowns. But my parents didn't know better; they had little help learning about their ND daughter. But today, we can know better for our kids. We can accept them for who they are and teach them how to accept themselves.

Deirdre Atkinson-Byrne, an Australian neurodiversity advocate who wasn't diagnosed with autism until she was an adult, grew up with parents who affirmed her feelings during the holidays despite her lack of diagnosis. She writes, describing opening holiday gifts, "If I didn't like it, I would say 'Thanks Mam, but I don't like the colour of this, I'm going to take it back if that's ok?'" Her honesty during the holidays didn't create negative consequences. Importantly, she points out, "There was NO expectation to pretend, a.k.a. mask, my true feelings. My opinion was valued." Her parents accepted her and her siblings "for who we were."[33]

Atkinson-Byrne recognizes that her experience is not the norm. She once was given a social story to help preview Christmas for her own neurodivergent children, and, to her shock, it was supposed to teach kids "how to explicitly hide their own feelings about their gift in order to protect the gifter's feelings." She writes, "Did they understand that they were training their child to fawn, to put someone else's needs over their own? To suppress their true thoughts and feelings in order to be liked? Did they know they are teaching their autistic children and clients to mask?" Fawning, a behavior that many ND children develop, centers people-pleasing behavior to appease an aggressor (such as an angry adult if you are a child), temper conflict, and keep themselves safe.

The holidays are chaotic, as Atkinson-Byrne describes, and that chaos takes a toll on ND children: "They might be feeling dysregulated by all of the noise around them, there might be too many people chatting, glasses clinking, children screaming, paper ripping, Christmas carols playing, lights flashing, people laughing, and people taking photos and videos." Add the pressure to please gift-givers to all of that and it is not surprising that ND kids would melt down.

Atkinson-Byrne has advice for parents of ND kids to help relieve the pressure of gifts amid the dysregulating chaos of the holidays. First, "talk to [your kids] about what they want." Second, she says, set boundaries with family members on their behalf. For example, "say thank you on [your kid's] behalf and let them open them in private later." You, as a parent, might feel social pressure to have your kid open the gift in front of the giftgiver. But if your kid doesn't want to, don't make them. The gift is for the child, not for the ego of the giver. As you might imagine, this advice works well for *all* kids.

If we preview chaotic events to reduce the chaos, set boundaries, and give our kids the freedom to take breaks, we can often prevent emotional dysregulation—and therefore meltdowns—from happening in the first place. But as my family's trip to the animal shelter showed, ND families can't prepare for everything. Sometimes things just go sideways and get overwhelming, and there's nothing we can do about it. What then?

After Goldeneye was taken away from him at the animal shelter, I let my son cry all he wanted on a bench outside the shelter. I let him express all of his overwhelming emotions. I did not force my son to mask and hide his neurodivergent expression. By the time we got to the restaurant, he was disappointed, but after the emotional cleanse, he was okay. If we want *all* of our kids to grow up to be emotionally healthy adults, we will give them space to cry and feel their feelings, whether they are neurotypical or neurodivergent. I now see that I have rarely given myself the same leeway. When I stood at the checkout counter and was told that it was too late to adopt, the upswell of disappointment hit me hard. I tried to keep my own emotions clamped down tight. Some tears leaked out, and I immediately felt ashamed.

The next day, when I returned to the shelter to pick up Goldeneye, I still felt ashamed by the small slip in my mask from the day before. I worried that the woman at the counter would treat me with disdain for having lost control. That is how insidious the social shaming of neurodivergent emotional expression can be. Even under the aegis of the director of the shelter, I feared contempt. We must protect our children from this ableist contempt. They will come up against it, but that doesn't mean they must feel ashamed of who they are.

When our kids are young, we must protect them from the cruelty of others the way I protected my child at the shelter, the way Sophia protects her son, and the way Atkinson-Byrne suggests we protect our children at the holidays. We can preview. We can discuss with them the options they have to keep themselves safe—especially our children of color, who face an exponential risk of violence toward themselves from outsiders. We must make sure that our children feel free to express their emotions safely and know how to do so. We can speak up for our children if others tell them not to cry or to stop crying. We can acknowledge and affirm their tears. This affirmation can help *all* kids, not just ND kids.

Because our ND children will be judged for their emotions, we can help them learn about their emotions sooner and more deliberately than neurotypical kids might need to do. Our kids will need clear language to describe their emotions to the adults who have control over their lives, such as teachers and coaches. This ability to describe their emotions is known as "emotional literacy." Emotional literacy is composed of many skills, but the first one is "self-awareness" of one's emotions, which is "the skill which helps to label and name emotions."[34] Psychologists recognize that "the ability to label emotions is a developmental skill that is not present at birth—it must be learned."[35] Furthermore, "some children's ability to identify, understand, and label their emotions develops at a slower rate than others." Our ND kids will likely develop this skill more slowly because they tend to struggle with learning emotions solely from social cues. At the same time, they have a greater need of it because the world will give their emotional expressions less leeway. If they can communicate their emotions well, then they have another way of protecting themselves against shame.

How can we teach our young kids how to name their emotions? You can name your own emotions when you feel them and talk about ways that you handle them. When your kids are young, you can also name *their* emotions when they feel them: "You seem happy to play with that toy," for example. As they get older, you can collaborate on this naming: "Are you scared to ride the bus?" I used a tool with my children—a board game called Mixed Emotions.[36] The game board had a wealth of emotions named on it, grouped in color "zones," which we used as a shorthand: sad, happy, angry, worried. We still use this shorthand today, even though they're in their teens. I use it to talk about my own emotions with them, too.

As they grow older, we must teach our children how to express their emotions safely so that they aren't punished for doing so. We must teach them that if they feel a meltdown or shutdown coming on, expressing it is nothing to be ashamed of. But we must also teach them that many outsiders will punish them for the behavior and that sometimes that punishment can be dangerous or deadly. We must also teach them that mistreatment of ND people for their natural behavior is wrong and unjust.

As we teach our kids to protect themselves against public shaming, we must also teach them how to protect themselves from violence, such as violence from bullies, teachers, and, even worse, police—especially if you have a ND child of color. Encourage them to find a private place to melt down, such as a bathroom if they are in a public building or in their car if they're old enough to drive and have a vehicle. But always make sure to reinforce that their behavior is not wrong; the public response to it is.

And if they can't find a private place, you can give them some words to use to explain to others what they might be experiencing. For example, my son could say, "I am so disappointed about the cat that I'm going to cry about it. I'll be back in a little while." With practice, these words can create bubble of social safety for our kids.

The research conducted on the public shaming of parents and ND children tells us that we need to create not only "a greater awareness of the emotional complexity of public encounters" for parents but also "a greater understanding of the children's behaviour" for the public at large. Only by creating awareness and understanding will we create "more tolerance for unusual behaviours in public places."[37] But, in the face of glacial social change, how do we create this tolerance?

Neurodivergent adults who have the security (financial or social, for example) and the emotional bandwidth can help bring about change. We can say out loud what we are experiencing. In doing so, we can widen the scope of acceptable emotions. For example, if a store's sign is wrong, like the one at the animal shelter, we can say so out loud. And then, we can do what I failed to do that day when I suppressed my tears: We can share how the misinformation has affected us. I could have said, "Your information did not say anything about a thirty-minute limit. Now I am really frustrated." If you are crying in order to release that frustration, say, "My frustration is why I am crying." If it is safe to do so, you can even say out loud that you are neurodivergent and that their failures make their space inaccessible.

I recognize that being able to say these things and to demand acceptance is hard. Even identifying how you feel in the midst of a stressful emotional moment can be impossible. I also recognize that drawing attention to one's neurodivergence is something that a ND adult may not want to do for fear of being ostracized both by friends and family and in the workplace. Therefore, many ND adults will not be able to do what I've described, and that is okay. This is activist work, and there is no shame in avoiding it. Just living in the world as a neurodivergent person is difficult enough.

Years ago, I couldn't say any of these things at the animal shelter because I felt too ashamed of my tears; plus, I didn't know that I was autistic. I just thought I was made wrong. I'm not ashamed anymore, and an autism diagnosis plus therapy have helped me put that shame aside. Now, these are words I would say in order to create a better world for my children. In fact, in other contexts, I have said them.

As parents, we can learn how to be comfortable around different kinds of emotional expressions. We were all raised within a society with ableist social norms, and therefore we were also raised to enforce them. We have to take active steps to stop ourselves from shaming our ND children, otherwise we might do so without even realizing it. When we allow our children space to express all of their emotions safely, we are, indeed, changing the world.

CHAPTER 3

Masking, Treatments, and Affirming Neurodiversity

My kids are seven and nine, and my family is at a fancy resort in the Appalachians, a sprawling hotel built near ancient hot springs. We come in the summer for the swimming pools and the enormous acreage where we can let the kids explore without worrying about social surveillance of their behavior. My weird and wonderful family doesn't fit in very well with most of the other families here, but the resort grounds are so big that we have enough room to be ourselves.

Except for tonight. Because of a late-afternoon thunderstorm, the resort had to move a celebration barbecue indoors. Earlier, the crowd was small, but now it is growing and making me anxious. My older son, Nine, dances as a kid-oriented cover band plays "You're Welcome" from *Moana*. He's moving like he's the only person in the room. Every few moments, he turns and throws me a grin. I feel his joy as I take him in. But as people finish eating and the dance floor gets full, I feel uneasy and protective.

After a few songs, Nine runs up to the lead singer and requests a song by Imagine Dragons, his favorite band. It's an odd request given the Disney-heavy playlist of the evening; plus, no one else has made a request of the band. But Nine hasn't picked up on the social norms of this particular event, where, it appears, song requests aren't a *thing*.

His dancing doesn't match the social norms, either. Other kids his age are dancing in a group. But he dances alone, bouncing around the dance floor, only occasionally encountering the beat. No one could doubt that he has joy for the music. But as I watch him, I worry. His left arm drifts near a woman in a boat-necked sweater. His sneaker lands close to another dancer's boat shoe.

I catch his father's eye. *Please*, I say to my husband with a glance. *Please tell Nine to rein it in.* But then I halt myself. Is that really what I want? Do I really want Nine to dance stiff-armed, to be hemmed in by self-consciousness? No. That's what I've been trained to want for him. That's how I've been told he should behave by his old teachers before we left them behind to homeschool. By camp counselors who say he talks out of turn. By the piano teacher who dramatically quit after three lessons.

If I stop and think, if I set aside the judgmental glances from the woman in the cardigan and her friend in the designer flip-flops, then I know for certain that the last thing I want is for Nine to rein anything in.

I want him to let all of his exuberance fly. On the dance floor. Or when he's talking to strangers about dinosaurs and cats and his other special interests. Or when he's designing robots that his robot kit wasn't intended to make—the dog model will become a *Star Wars* AT-AT (those giant walkers on the snow planet Hoth), whether it was meant to be or not.

As his mother, it's not my job to make him smaller so he can fit into rigid social norms. No. My job is to make the world larger: to find bigger dance floors, to find people willing to listen to his ideas, to find more robust robot kits. And to let him dance how he likes. It's dancing, after all. Nine's capaciousness is not the problem. Finding a world big enough for him, however, can be a serious challenge as his mom.

As I watched him dance, I feared something tangible, however. Not the social ostracization that I would experience as his mom but that he would experience as a neurodivergent kid. I know what he'll experience because I experienced it myself. My initial desire to rein him in wasn't to make him normal for normal's sake but to protect him from the painful mockery I experienced as a kid.

Fighting against my own internalized ableism and awful childhood memories, I've resisted telling my children to rein it in. Instead, I've given them unconditional love and stories about how the world treats people like us so that they can make informed decisions. Today, my older son is fifteen, and he's grown up to be self-assured, self-possessed, and socially bulletproof. It *can* happen. But it took an immense leap of faith on my part, handing him knowledge about ableism and then stepping back and letting him use it how he sees fit.

When I was nine, I was also boisterous and socially oblivious. My obliviousness didn't go away as I turned ten, then eleven, finishing elementary school and entering middle school. No one helped me understand that I wasn't made wrong. Instead, they did the opposite.

My mother used to talk to me about my deficiency in "social skills"—her phrase. Her tone was usually exasperated and sometimes, to my young ears, mean. To this day, even in my forties, when I hear the phrase "social skills" I want to curl into a ball and protect my soft middle. But when I was nine, ten, fifteen, sixteen, my mother didn't have all of the information that I have now. I wasn't diagnosed neurodivergent as a child. Girls were frequently overlooked by doctors back then because there was, and still is, a strong diagnostic bias toward white boys.[1] Because of this bias, I am part of the "lost generation" of adults whose autism went undiagnosed when we were children.[2] A diagnosis might have helped my mother realize that although I appeared physically older than my age, and although I was intellectually advanced for my age, I was decidedly *not* socially on par for my age. Quite the opposite. I was socially immature because of my undiagnosed autism, and that immaturity made me vulnerable.

At the same time, a diagnosis might not have helped at all. Few, if any, therapies for autism were neurodiversity affirming when I was a kid. Applied Behavior Analysis (ABA) therapy dominated autism treatment at the time and arguably still does.[3] If I had been put into ABA therapy as a child, it would have trained me to stifle my differences, to act more in line with social norms, and to believe that being autistic is a flaw to be fixed.[4] I wouldn't have thrived in a treatment like that. I would have rebelled, or I would have crumpled. Probably a little bit of both.

Instead, I was on my own. When I was eleven—starting sixth grade—I appeared thirteen, could read and talk like I was sixteen, and acted eight or nine. On the first day of middle school, after a long summer apart, I ran up to my best friend in the lunch line. I was so happy to see her that I couldn't contain my joy. And why would I?

I said to her, "Do you want to come over and play after school?"

She looked at me, uncertain. The other girls around us laughed. I didn't know why, not until later, when my friend explained to me in private, "We don't *play* anymore. We *hang out.*"

I'd embarrassed her, I realized. And I'd embarrassed myself. For the first time, I felt the knife of my own social wrongness. I was not alone in my struggle to bridge the vast social gulf between elementary and middle school. Research shows that social systems grow more numerous and complex as kids move from elementary to middle school, and these social systems make life difficult for autistic girls.[5]

I've never forgotten how hard it was to fit in as a child, to do it so poorly and with so little help. Because I made good grades and didn't act out at school (at least not for a few more years), I didn't receive support for the bullying I experienced or the internal pain I felt when I tried to fit in.

But I want to be able to help my kids. Like my kids, I was always the last one to get the joke. I was always afraid at the scary movies. I always had the worst "social skills." I don't blame my mom for being frustrated—she didn't know any better. But I refuse to be angry at my children. They're doing nothing except being who they are.

I'm lucky that I had the experiences I did so that I can better help my kids. I know what it's like to be the one who dances weird. I know what it's like to feel the crushing weight of self-awareness when it hits. I refuse to force that self-awareness on my kids. I know it will come soon enough, but it will not come from me. No, I've been there to help them through it and remind them that it is the world that is wrong, not them. It is my job to affirm their neurodiversity. To prevent internalized ableism so that they can grow into themselves and understand that who they are is perfectly imperfect, just like a human is supposed to be.

So on that dance floor in the mountains, I reminded myself how much I love Nine's dancing. He is an energized particle, shedding love and joy. I thought of the dance parties we have at home, when I played Nine's favorite songs and our family danced all over the kitchen, the four of us: Nine and his little brother, Seven, bouncing around each other while their father and I danced together like we did when we first met—a little bit of swing, a little bit of cha-cha-cha. At the resort that afternoon, my husband and I spread our arms wide to make room for Nine. Together, we created a place where Nine could safely carom to the music. *Here*, I thought. *You have space here, for now.*

Later, I promised myself, I would make sure he learns how to make space for himself.

MASKING

When I mention the "crushing weight of self-awareness," I'm referring to the realization that how you act, what you do—*who you are*—as a neurodivergent person is somehow inherently wrong and shameful. Neurodivergent people are ostracized simply for existing.[6] Narrow, ableist social norms punish ND people for existing outside of them. This punishment of ND kids starts far earlier than we think, and it doesn't hit all at once. Often it starts when other kids bully ND kids, recognizing them as targets. Neurodivergent kids are at a much higher risk of bullying than neurotypical kids are, at a rate of 67 percent, according to a recent study.[7] But all of us, even ND people, play a role in enforcing social norms because of our own internalized ableism. It is impossible to live in our society and not internalize bigotry against ND people. It is too pervasive.

For example, media portrayals of neurodivergent characters who step outside of social norms reinforce how wrong it is to do so by showing their punishment on screen. On *The Big Bang Theory*, the autistic character Sheldon is never good enough, even for his friends.[8] His friends mock him, yell at him, and express their wish that he would change. He rarely finds acceptance for who he is. Although the showrunners never state outright that Sheldon is autistic, he is strongly coded as such. This coding of characters as ND, rather than naming them so, is common. Imagine how different the show would have been if Sheldon had understood his autism and how it affected his life. There would have been far fewer jokes because the show's humor relied on his ignorance of his autism. It is difficult to watch a neurodivergent character be so mistreated by the people who are supposed to love him, especially on one of the most popular television shows ever made—it ran for twelve seasons, and a prequel series with similar tropes, *Young Sheldon*, ran through 2024. It is especially hard to watch when you know that media portrayals of the mistreatment of ND people justify such mistreatment in real life.

On the show *Hannibal*, the main character, Will Graham, states almost plainly that he is autistic in the first episode, when an FBI agent is recruiting him to help with a crime scene.[9] The agent says, "I understand that it's difficult for you to be social. Where do you fall on the spectrum?" Graham replies that he is "closer to Asperger's and autistics." Graham's odd behavior causes many of his colleagues to mistrust him. Later, he becomes (or is revealed to be) a murderer and a sociopath. Portrayals of sociopathic "autistic" people contribute to the false stereotype that autistic people are more violent than neurotypical people.[10] In reality, it is autistic people who experience victimization at an alarming rate.[11]

Some shows do a better job not only accurately portraying neurodivergent characters but also showing them in relationships with people who love them just as they are. One example, on the TV show *Community*, is Abed Nadir, who is heavily coded as autistic.[12] In an op-ed, late-diagnosed autistic disability studies scholar (and then-undergraduate) Kate Ellis writes, "I immediately connected with Abed. This was a character that got me—I watched him dump his life story on Jeff before he even introduced himself in the pilot episode, and it was like seeing myself on television in the best and most confusing way." But, unlike Sheldon's friends on *The Big Bang Theory*, as Ellis points out, "Abed's friends accept and encourage his interests, instead of making fun of them."[13] However, Abed's character is the exception, not the norm.

Because of the mistreatment and social ostracization neurodivergent people experience, we learn to hide our differences. We hide them to avoid making others uncomfortable and also to protect ourselves from harm. This hiding is commonly called "masking," and psychologists also call it "camouflaging."[14] According to psychologists, writing in the context of autism, "Camouflaging refers to the behavior of using coping strategies in social situations to hide behaviors associated with ASD [autism], through the use of explicit techniques to seem socially proficient, and through attempts to prevent others from seeing their social difficulties."[15] ND people mask in order to fit in socially, hoping that it will make our lives easier. Masking is often effective in hiding ND traits, but it comes with a cost. Psychologists note that it is "cognitively effortful and taxing; prone to breakdown under increased social demands and complexity and/or psychological distress; and associated with increased mental health difficulties."[16]

Masking is commonly done unconsciously. Psychologist Devon Price writes, in their book *Unmasking Autism*, that masking begins as soon as autistic people take our first breath: "Autistic people are born with a mask of neurotypicality pressed against our faces."[17] At a young age, ND children internalize the knowledge that masking protects us by hiding who we are, and the habit of masking becomes ingrained. As Price writes, "When an Autistic person is not given resources or access to self-knowledge, and when they're told their stigmatized traits are just signs that they're a disruptive, overly sensitive, or annoying kid, they have no choice but to develop a neurotypical facade."[18] Masking extends beyond autistics to any neurodivergent people who act in ways that are stigmatized by neurotypical society.

For many neurodivergent people, ableism and stigma force them to keep masking because being their true selves would mean losing their job or friends. So although being neurodivergent is a normal way to be human, one with strengths as well as struggles, as Devon Price has pointed out, ableism can cause "incredible alienation and pain."[19] Because of this pain, ND people mask. We mask because the people we spend our time with do not affirm neurodiversity. Instead, because of social norms, ND people, even kids, are shamed for being different—for simply being themselves.

STIMMING

When I was in preschool, a group of parents kicked me out of our preschool carpool because I wouldn't sit quietly or stand still. Behaviors such as these can be boiled down to one: "fidgeting." Fidgeting, in the context of ND kids, is one type of "self-stimulatory behavior" (as psychologists call it), or "stimming" (as ND people call it).[20] Stimming by ND people "involve[s] repetitive movements or sounds" that sometimes go beyond the barriers of social norms.[21] Neurotypical people stim: Foot tapping is stimming, and so is fiddling with a pen. This stimming is socially acceptable. Some stimming by ND people, however, such as pacing, rocking, noisemaking, or hand flapping, can go beyond the acceptable.

Stimming serves an important purpose for the psychological health of ND people: It can help ND people cope with anxiety caused by overstimulation, distressing situations, and uncertainty (like last-minute changes in plans).[22] A subtype of stimming, called "distress stimming," is a way that a ND person can communicate that they are hurting in some way. *All* stimming is communication, though. If a person is stimming, they need to do it, and if they need to do it, there's a reason why.

When we look at the connection between stimming and anxiety, we must look at how common anxiety is in ND kids. Research shows that it is a common co-neurodivergence in autistic and ADHD kids.[23] Common anxiety sources among these kids "included being rejected, letting people down, being different, having no friends, or being punished for getting things wrong." For ADHDers, research has shown that the negative feedback that children receive from those around them due to their ADHD expression can itself cause anxiety.[24] In addition, research shows that some executive function struggles that come along with ADHD, such as emotional regulation, can reduce a child's ability to deal with stressful situations, increasing their anxiety over time.

With anxiety being so frequently a part of a ND kid's life, stimming becomes essential for the health of our children because it soothes that anxiety. But stimming has been misunderstood by researchers and doctors for decades and often continues to be. Adults with autism and other neurodivergences are now speaking out about the importance of stimming to their health. These adults are a wonderful resource for parents of ND kids because we can learn from them how to help our kids understand what stimming is and that it is normal and healthy. We can also learn to avoid the ineffectual and harmful "treatment" offered by some therapists to "extinguish self-stimulation behaviors" in ND children.[25] When therapists try to suppress stimming, they suppress the tools a ND person needs to self-regulate and/or communicate their emotions. A child whose stimming has been suppressed will find another way to communicate their distress, such as through meltdowns, breakdowns, or self-harm.[26]

One parent I interviewed, Sophia, has a teenaged son who is AuDHD. A white woman who lives in the South, she describes her family as "pro-safe-stimming."[27] Sophia makes sure that her son understands that stimming is a fine thing to do: "I reassure him that it is okay to stim." She also takes into account the needs of her son to stim alongside the needs of others in public. She told me, "There is the very real pressure of balancing what my son needs or wants with the needs of others. Because it's one thing to say, 'My son needs to stim in public.' But when that stimming is infringing on other people's needs, there's a lot of pressure in being the parent and balancing that out." Sophia is a good model for how to balance her son's stimming needs and those of the larger world. She explained, "He has a high voltage energy sometimes. And I say, 'Okay, I understand that you feel like you need to climb up on this picnic table and jump around and leap off it. But other people have needs, and their needs are not having your shoes around where their food is.'" But it is hard work helping her son find and understand this balance: "Along with that [balancing] is a hypervigilance of knowing that you have to keep an eye out for these moments when you need to balance things."

In order to help her son find safe ways to stim in public, Sophia presents him with alternatives that we, as parents, can also learn from: "All kids are different. Obviously, this is going to be different for different kids. My kid loves going to restaurants, loves going out to eat. But during those minutes between ordering and the food coming, we go outside, take a little walk." In other words, she doesn't demand her son sit quietly at the table and wait for his food. She lets him express his excitement

and impatience outside. Her son understands that going outside is not a punishment but rather a way to safely stim in public. In this way, she is honest with him about stimming and also
affirms it.

Sophia always asks if anything is stressing out her son and
causing the stimming because, for ND kids, that is often the
case. She told me, "I say, 'Hey, you're stimming a lot. Are you getting agitated? Do you need a break?' He's usually able to say,
'Yes, I need a break,' and then we take a break. We leave. We go
outside." Sophia explained how she reassures her son that the
need to stim is fine: "While reassuring him that, 'Okay, you need
to do some stimming, fine. I understand. But let's find a different space or an alternative, something else to do.' Or I remove
the thing that might be agitating."

Fidgeting—stimming—is one way all human bodies handle
difficult emotions. Think of a room full of children. Are they sitting still? No, because *all* kids fidget, especially when they are
in some kind of distress: overstimulated, tired, anxious, or
bored. But fidgeting by ND kids may seem more extreme than
fidgeting by neurotypical kids. Or, in stressful situations, ND
kids may begin fidgeting sooner than neurotypical kids will, as
they are more sensitive to the environment. My message to any
teachers, coaches, counselors, or parents is that, if a ND kid (or
adult) starts fidgeting, figure out why and improve conditions
in your classroom / camp / team practice / home. Otherwise,
your neurotypical kids will soon follow. Neurodivergent people
are like canaries in the overstimulating coal mine.

The best way to cope with stimming—your own or that of
someone you love—is through acceptance, as Sophia demonstrated.[28] Medical research shows that stimming only needs
treatment when it causes harm to the ND person or those
around them, such as hitting oneself or others.[29] If you are a

parent worried about your child's stimming, take a step back. In what context did the stimming arise? Look for the distress that may have caused the stimming in the first place. And if it is caused by joy, rather than distress, then celebrate with them.

CURES FOR DESPERATE PARENTS

First, I want to say this: We are here, making the journey through this book together, because we want to do what is best for our children. But we must also acknowledge that sometimes figuring out what is best for our kids can be really, really hard. I have made mistakes along the way, some of which I deeply regret. Perhaps you have too. One of the biggest challenges that we face is an invisible one: the pressure that our society places on us to mold our children to fit into a narrow set of norms because they will be ostracized or even physically harmed if they don't.

Desperate, well-meaning parents of ND kids are frequently sold the lie that if their kid can be forced into behaving in a neurotypical fashion, then their kid will be happier and safer. Being "normal" seems like an escape from bullying and so forth, right? But the truth is that accepting and embracing a kid's neurodivergence is the best protection we can give them against a hostile world. With greater self-understanding, ND kids become more self-assured.[30] Our job as parents is to unlink neurodivergence from shame—that is, to be neurodiversity affirming. But figuring out how to parent in a way that affirms neurodiversity can be really hard.

It is true that the behavior of neurodivergent kids frequently does not comply with narrow social norms. Research shows that when parents of ND children are in public, they face public shaming when their kids' behavior violates social norms.[31] The good news is that this same research (and my own) shows that parents felt no shame toward their children or their autistic identities and behaviors. Instead, they were empathetic with their kids and struggled only with the judgmental outsiders. Nevertheless, parents want to protect their children, and this desire to protect makes them vulnerable to bad parenting advice, bad medical advice, and even dangerous advice.

School is one place where this bad advice lands on us like an avalanche. Like many parents of ND kids, I was vulnerable when my kids first started school. It felt like they did everything wrong—because the school told me that they did. During an awful parent-teacher conference with my younger child's kindergarten teacher, among other things, the teacher told me that my son couldn't follow the "morning tasks" list properly, in which the students were to take off coats, put away lunches, get their notebooks, and so on, and so forth, in the order she expected. She also told me that my son hid under the table and "refused" to come out. (I recount this story in more detail in the introduction.) After half an hour of hearing about his terrible behavior (in the teacher's eyes), I blurted out to her that I was having him tested for ADHD and that he would be starting medication soon.

My words were the truth, but my motives feel shameful to me now. I shared this private medical information to appease the teacher, not to form a collaboration with her. She didn't care about his neurodiversity. She only wanted him to behave neurotypically and, with my words, I assured her that I was going to make that happen. The horrible part is that my words worked; she was indeed appeased, sniffing and nodding like a queen toward a supplicant. Because I was afraid of the teacher, I betrayed my kid's privacy in order to assuage her. In retrospect, she was a bully, and I folded under her bullying. The only thing that saves me from being too hard on myself today is that I made the right choice in testing my kids for ADHD and that supportive therapy and medication have really helped them.

I'm not alone in feeling bullied by schools to change my kids' behavior. In her book *Your Child Is Not Broken*, neurodivergent author Heidi Mavir recounts a story of her ND kid's suffering at the hands of his school when they, too, tried to make him more neurotypical. After her son was labeled a "school refuser" because he would melt down when it came time to go to school (not unlike my kid shutting down and hiding under his desk), the special education coordinator (SEC) assigned to him gave Heidi and her son a task: Heidi had to drive her son to school. Then, he had to touch the school gate so that he wouldn't be counted absent. Despite her reservations, Mavir agreed to this plan. She describes the SEC's response to her agreement, "Susi gave a triumphant nod. For a moment, I wondered if she might be about to give me a reward sticker in recognition of my being so compliant."[32] Mavir points out that "school refusal" is a fake label. She calls it "a bullshit piece of parent- and child-blaming to draw focus away from the fact that a child is struggling and probably has unmet needs."[33] Social pressures that parents face to make our kids seem neurotypical are tough. Mavir, myself, and parents that I've interviewed describe caving to the demands of schools and other authority figures who demand neurotypicality because they believe the others know what's best for ND kids. (They do not.)

Because of social pressure to conform, some parents use treatments that are harmful, even if they don't realize it. Among the fake treatments for autism, for example, is Miracle Mineral Solution (MMS), composed of chlorine dioxide, a bleaching compound parents feed their children, use as an enema, or put in bathwater.[34] The theory behind MMS treatment is that the bleach kills the pathogens that cause autism in the body.[35] But autism is not caused by pathogens, and bleach destroys the soft tissue of the digestive system.

Another fake cure for autism is chelation therapy, which circulates a chemical through the bloodstream to remove toxic chemicals such as mercury. Chelation therapy is appealing because some parents still incorrectly believe that autism is caused by mercury in childhood vaccines—a myth created by a scientist named Andrew Wakefield in the 1990s and since debunked by everyone in the scientific community.[36] However, the myth still holds sway among some parents. These parents are sold the lie that chelation will cure autism. But although chelation is an actual medical treatment for poisoning, for example, it comes with risks that include kidney damage and heart failure.

Other cures include severely modified diets or added supplements. One common danger posed by these cures is financial ruin, as parents spend vast amounts of money on special foods and supplements. However, physical dangers exist as well—children can suffer nutrient imbalances from food-elimination diets (intended to figure out which foods are causing autistic traits) and react badly to supplements. Another treatment is hyperbaric therapy, in which children are exposed to higher-than-normal levels of oxygen and air pressure in order to treat "damage and inflammation in the brain," according to one hyperbaric center that claims to treat autism.[37] Hyperbaric therapy is expensive, with the treatment providers requiring dozens of sessions for treatment to be successful. A review of the research has shown that the treatment does not have any benefits.[38]

These false treatments gain traction because ableism tells us that all ND kids need to be "fixed." But not only do the treatments cause physical harm to children, they also wipe out parental funds.

WHAT ABOUT ABA?

In this discussion of cures, I have so far evaded the elephant in the room, the so-called gold standard (at least in the United States) for treating autism and other similar neurodivergences. I'm referring to Applied Behavior Analysis. ABA is the therapy endorsed by Autism Speaks, one of the largest autism nonprofits in the world. ABA has been endorsed by family doctors and courts of law.[39] In the United States, state-level mandates ensure that private insurance companies cover the cost of ABA.[40] If a doctor prescribes ABA for a child, then Medicaid must cover the treatment. In fact, for most medical insurance companies, ABA is the only autism treatment that they will cover at all.[41]

Frequently, parents with newly diagnosed ND kids are told by doctors that ABA is their only option. In her book *I Will Die on This Hill* (coauthored with autistic adult Jules Edwards), author Meghan Ashburn, mother of autistic children, tells how ABA was pushed on her by her doctor.[42] After telling Ashburn that her toddler was autistic, the doctor handed her a folder and said, "The standard treatment is ABA (applied behavioral analysis). I put a script and a list of providers in the folder. You'll want to get started right away." She continues, "Those were basically the only things he put in that folder, aside from a useless single-page printout about what autism is." Later, when Ashburn pushed back about other treatment options, "the only treatment he recommended was ABA. Full stop." When parents who are facing a new and intimidating diagnosis are given a singular path—ABA—by the doctor who is caring for their kid, then it isn't surprising when they choose that singular path.

Autism Speaks describes the goal of ABA as "to increase behaviors that are helpful and decrease behaviors that are harmful or affect learning."[43] In other words, ABA is a "behavior therapy, not a cognitive or emotional one," keyed to making a ND kid less disruptive to neurotypical norms.[44] ABA is a type of "compliance-based" behavior modification therapy. It uses punishments and rewards to train ND kids to behave in a way that is acceptable in a neurotypical society.

The problem is, such a strong focus on behavior leaves little room for care of the emotional well-being of the child. Recently, via email, I interviewed pediatric speech and language pathologist Jessie Mewshaw, an ADHDer who is also a parent of two neurodivergent kids.[45] Simply put, behavior modification therapies such as ABA require a child to perform a task, and then the child receives a reward for complying. As Mewshaw explained, a behavior modification treatment is "any attempt to modify or change the child in order to make the people around the child more comfortable." Behavior modification therapies "are not actually focused on the child's comfort and actually helping the child to become self-actualized and their authentic self." Instead, "it's all about the (primarily) neurotypical people around the child experiencing discomfort because of them."

For example, meltdowns are an expression of the emotional dysregulation of the child (or adult). ABA aims to halt meltdowns with aversive punishments or with rewards, focusing solely on the behavior (the meltdown). Compare this approach with neurodiversity-affirming (neuroaffirming) approaches, where the goal may be to figure out what is causing the dysregulation in the first place (itchy clothes? loud noises?) and teaching the kid about their emotions and tools to help them self-regulate. Conversely, behavior modification therapy makes the child compliant to adult demands and teaches them to ignore their own needs.

If you lift the cover off ABA, you'll find a few alarming facts. First, it was created in 1961 by Dr. Ole Ivar Lovaas "to condition neurotypical behaviors in children he viewed as 'incomplete humans.'"[46] Lovaas also created antigay conversion therapy, which similarly taught young people to suppress their own needs—and was ineffective.[47] Then, for decades, ABA therapists punished children by using electroshock devices and other painful negative reinforcements. These "aversives" were endorsed by ABA's governing body, the Association for Behavior Analysis International (ABAI), and were only rejected by the ABAI in 2022.[48] Psychological research has shown that ABA causes posttraumatic symptoms in its clients.[49] Other studies show that it is ineffective.[50] Therapists who work with ND children agree.[51] Studies by government bodies who pay for ABA, such as the military's Tricare insurance, show that ABA is ineffective in nearly 90 percent of cases.[52] And in 2023, the American Medical Association (AMA) removed its endorsement of ABA for many reasons, including that "modern ABA still abides by the founding principle of making a child appear 'normal' or 'indistinguishable from one's peers,' which serves to separate the humanity of the individual with autism from desired behaviors."[53]

In the face of this criticism, the ABA community has launched a public-image campaign. In response to the research showing the harm caused by ABA and its ineffectiveness, fierce ABA proponents have tried to debunk these claims with publications of their own. But their arguments are rarely based on original research and instead on attempts to poke holes in existing research critical of ABA.[54] They argue, in both professional and popular publications, that ABA's self-governance is strong enough to prevent abuse.

Another common defense by ABA professionals is that only "bad ABA" causes trauma.[55] ABA proponents acknowledge that "bad ABA" is out there and that it is indeed harmful. One therapy website's description of "good ABA" includes this parental testimony about their child: "He will focus more on tasks, particularly with the type of behavior plan that we have with him where he knows that first he has to do his task and then he gets to do his fun thing or get his reward."[56] But this task-reward system held up as good ABA remains the same type of behavior modification training that is at the heart of ABA, teaching children to obey without question or without understanding the context of what they are doing.

One parent I interviewed, however, shared that ABA has been the most effective therapy for her child. Cameron, a Black woman who is the mother of a twice-exceptional six-year-old autistic son, told me, "I love ABA therapy. I know that it gets mixed reviews. It's worked for us."[57] When her son's pre-K program failed him, Cameron told me, they went "full force" with ABA, speech therapy, and occupational therapy. She praised ABA for how much it has helped her child and told me his success stories. Her son, she told me, "loves to play and pretend. . . . [ABA] taught him how to play with cars. He loves cars, and he would just look at car books, but he didn't really understand, 'Oh, you can take the cars. You can make scenarios.'" When her son is with his therapist, "all they do is play. Like, 'Let's race cars,' and [the therapist] teaches [him] how to make the sounds, and [he] comes home and he does it." During the course of our interview, she did not describe any compliance-based rewards or punishments. Indeed, the collaborative play therapy that Cameron described in our interview sounds like it could be affirming, rather than behavior modification.

While some people argue that ABA can never be neuroaffirming because of its basis in compliance, some ABA service providers insist that what Cameron described is the type of ABA they provide.[58] One practice describes their approach in a way that sounds similar: "We aim to make everyone feel safe and valued, ensuring that our approach is tailored to meet unique needs and foster resilience, collaboration, and empowerment. It's about building a space where families can thrive together, understanding each person's unique journey and providing the right support along the way." However, the word "resilience" is a red flag. As Mavir puts it, "'Building Resilience' is professional-speak for behavior modification."[59] The idea, as Mavir relates in the context of her own son, is "to expand [her child's] window of tolerance to stimulus (in this case, school) so that he could respond to that stimulus in a more 'appropriate' way—in this case, by not becoming upset and refusing to go into the school building." But, as Mavir points out, behavior modification sought to "suppress his natural responses to something that was causing him harm." And suppressing natural responses in ND kids like Mavir's son, like mine and yours, only teaches them to "mask" those responses, to hide them so they can seem more neurotypical.

The point is, ABA has become fuzzy at its margins. If insurance will only cover ABA therapy, I can imagine that neuroaffirming therapists may put themselves under the ABA umbrella. Good for them. So long as insurance fails to cover other therapies, I support any method of providing care to ND kids, especially for families who can't afford to pay out of pocket. Good care should not be limited to the wealthy. Let us just ensure that what you select is indeed neuroaffirming.

THE SCHISM BETWEEN PARENTS
AND ND ADULTS

The behavior modification therapy debate brings to light a schism—and not just one between parents of neurodivergent kids. On one side of this schism are neurotypical parents of

autistic or other neurodivergent children who believe that behavior modification treatments are best. On the other side you
have autistic and other neurodivergent adults who believe that
any "treatment" that suppresses ND behavior is abusive. As autistic author C. L. Lynch writes, parents of ND kids and ND
adults "disagree on virtually everything, but arguably the most
contentious subject is Applied Behaviour Analysis Therapy."[60]
ABA and other behavior modification therapies are not only
used with autistic kids but with other neurodivergent kids as
well, such as kids with ADHD and more.

One of the arguments that parents of ND kids make about
the ABA schism is this: The ND adults speaking out against
ABA do not understand what it is like to be the parent of a ND
kid, especially one with high support needs. One pro-ABA parent interviewed about the ABA schism stated that "she understands the anti-ABA argument, but she wonders how much the
perspective of those who don't need a lot of support applies to
her son."[61] In other words, her son needs a lot of support, and
she presumes that the anti-ABA argument comes from the perspective of ND adults who did not need a lot of support as
children and who do not need it as adults. Her assumption re-
veals another aspect of the schism: ND parents presume that
the ND adults who speak out against behavior modification
treatments do not or did not have similar support needs as their
children do.

But the presumption that a ND adult who can write an Instagram post condemning certain treatments does not have high
support needs is inaccurate. Many ND advocates and authors
do have support needs that are greater than their adversaries
imagine. Some are nonspeaking, for example. Others cannot
drive. Furthermore, dismissing a person's opinion because of
their apparent support needs profile is harmful. Unfortunately,

this is common, as disability studies professor Jordynn Jack points out, writing, "Autistic individuals may actually be dismissed as too high-functioning, as 'shiny Aspies' unable to speak for or understand 'low-functioning' autistics."[62] We now know that support needs do not flow in a straight line but rather are "spiky," where a person might have high needs in one area and low needs in another. Ignoring a ND adult's voice because they're not "neurodivergent enough" does damage to what could be an immense collaboration. However, rampant criticism of parenting by ND people does the same.

But stepping back, way back, we can see that the schism isn't caused by ND parents or ND adults. It is caused by social pressures put on parents that drive them to seek treatment for their kids in the first place (applied by, for example, doctors or schools), by the lobbies for the organizations that pushed for insurance coverage for their treatments, and by the lack of a social safety net for ND people. Without a social safety net in place, a parent might believe—often rightly—that it would be easier for their kid to behave in a neurotypical fashion because they will avoid suffering. Our society does not provide adequate schooling or health care to neurodivergent people; ND people end up earning less and attaining less education. As a parent of a ND kid, these facts scare me.

All of us, on both sides of the behavior modification schism, must take on faith that the vast majority of parents want their kids to be happy. Social norms tell us that being different means being miserable. These norms are a powerful influence on all of us, including parents. If behavior modification therapy means a child will be more "normal," it must mean the child will be happier, right? For parents to navigate these complexities without help is difficult, and most parents do not have help. When ABA is the only therapy that most for-profit and public insurance will cover, parents are pressured by not only the government but also by some of the most powerful companies in the world to believe that behavior modification therapy is the only path forward.

Thus, the roots of the behavior modification therapy schism are institutional and societal pressures, not individual actions. These pressures pit ND adults and parents of ND kids against one another. Parents do not have a wealth of options to help their kids, unless they are financially able to pay out of pocket. If you lack funds, and the state or your insurance hands you an abundance of a particular free therapy for your child, you take it.

Emmy Award–winning neurodivergent comedian Hannah Gadsby writes a thoughtful message in their memoir directly to these parents, addressing the parents' concerns. Gadsby points out the low-grade hostility from parents that they have faced since sharing their autism diagnosis:

> Since making my [autism] diagnosis public, I have had some parents of nonverbal folk take me to task for identifying as autistic while not being as "disabled" as their child. To those people, I would like to say, I get it. I understand your frustration. It is my bet that you are not supported well enough, and that I seem like a good person to vent at. I don't mind. I can take it. But if it helps, it is not my intention to take anything away from you or your experience. All I want to do is help create something of a window into the inner workings of a manually processing brain. You know as well as I do that no two experiences are the same on the so-called spectrum; but I do know something of how frustrating and painfully lonely it can be from the inside. Ultimately we are on the same team.[63]

Gadsby insists we are on the same team, and we are. But I do know, as a ND parent who was once a ND kid, that it can be hard to see it. As Lynch writes, while autistic adults who have experienced ABA call it abusive, "you can imagine how that statement sounds to loving parents whose children adore their ABA therapist and who would never knowingly abuse their beloved child."[64] If you call a treatment abusive, you are calling the parent abusive. There is no beating around that bush.

So I want to say here, now, to all readers of this book: Whatever choices you have made, I am not here to judge you. I am only here to share with you my experiences and my research. I encourage you to follow my research and read the sources I cite and then do research of your own. I encourage all of us to keep an open mind. I hope this book can start mending this schism. You would not be reading this book if you didn't want to do the very best by your kid. I believe you do. I know you do.

AFFIRMING NEURODIVERSITY

Neurodiversity-affirming (or "neuroaffirming") care refers to therapy that does not view neurodivergence as something to be corrected but rather as a normal part of human diversity with strengths to be embraced. At the same time, neuroaffirming therapy recognizes the disabling aspects of a client's neurodivergence and collaborates with the client to find the best way to treat these aspects. Neuroaffirming therapy therefore helps ND kids learn to embrace their neurodivergences and does not require neurodivergent kids to mask their ND traits in order to appear more neurotypical. Meanwhile, it teaches them self-advocacy and boundaries, helping them learn the skills that the therapist and the client agree will help them live a fulfilling life.

According to pediatric speech and language pathologist Jessie Mewshaw, neuroaffirming care "very much centers the child's comfort and the child's authenticity and their self-advocacy skills, and it focuses on how they are going to grow up to be an adult human in the world."[65] Practically, this means taking into account the kid's needs and collaborating with the kid, and the parents, about what is best for the kid. Mewshaw is describing what is called "child-led therapy," which is "interest-based," and its goal is to bring "great passion and great joy" to the therapy sessions and the therapeutic relationship. But just because it is led by the child does not mean there aren't therapeutic goals. Mewshaw explains that a therapist does this work "while also honoring and embedding the goals created for that child, with the child as well as with the child's caregivers." As Mewshaw explains, "Collaboration and problem-solving are huge themes" in neuroaffirming therapy.

Sometimes therapy means recognizing that a kid is not ready for therapy when they enter the room. Mewshaw told me, "If they're coming in right after school," there might have been a lot of demands made on the kid that day. She says, "Sometimes I can see it as they're walking in the door because I'm very tuned to their nervous systems. I can tell just by the way that they're holding their body." So what's the problem? "If they're coming in semi-activated, that is not a good time for me to immediately put a demand on them by asking them a question." Why not? By putting demands on a kid who has already faced a lot of demands, you risk dysregulation.

Instead, Mewshaw explains, "My goal is, how do I get you back to a place of regulation and feeling social and safe, not to place demands that could then potentially trigger you into a meltdown." Mewshaw, as a neuroaffirming therapist, recognizes that the source of a meltdown is sensory or emotional overload. Meltdowns aren't tantrums to be squashed with punishments. They are a signal that the kid (or adult) has been made so uncomfortable that they can't take any more stimulation. It is her job to step back and figure out what led to the meltdown or to "co-regulate" with the kid and help them learn how to regulate their emotions as they grow older and more capable of doing so. She points out, "I cannot keep my own nervous system regulated every day throughout the day. Why would a child be able to do that?"

One of the goals of neuroaffirming care is for a child to always want to go to therapy. They should be excited to go, and they should trust their therapist. Mewshaw explained that her goal is to become a "safe adult" for the children she works with. She told me that if you have a ND kid or any kid, "the more safe people you can get in your little safe people Rolodex, the better."

PUSHING BACK AGAINST NORMS

Inclusion of neurodiversity in our society means accepting ND emotional expressions and understanding the causes of them, which will allow ND kids to avoid learning to mask. If we could eradicate neurodivergent masking, ND mental health would improve dramatically. But we're not there yet. Now, when a ND kid sobs over a disappointment in a toy store, a neurotypical person might perceive the kid as having a childish temper tantrum because the ND kid is expressing emotions in a fashion that is outside the bounds of current social norms. This lack of understanding causes harm, including "barriers to [ND families'] acceptance in public places," as research has shown, because parents in the study didn't want to subject their children to shaming by other adults.[66]

This narrow scope of acceptable emotional expression in neurotypical society harms all people who need to express emotions beyond the limits that our society permits our gender, our race, or any intersection thereof. Girls shouldn't be interested in trains (instead of, say, dolls) because social norms dictate that women are supposed to be nurturing. Boys shouldn't cry while having a meltdown because it offends traditional norms of masculinity.

Neurodivergent people of color face challenges that white people will never be able to comprehend (although we should do all we can to learn). Black women must avoid expressions of anger or high emotion to avoid being stereotyped as an "angry Black woman," which can put her schooling, career, or even life in danger. Black men face dangers if they melt down because strong emotional expressions are perceived as threatening by our society as a whole and law enforcement in particular. Research confirms that Black people in the US are *three times* more likely to die by police violence than white people.[67] As autistic author and activist Kala Allen Omeiza writes, "To be a Black autistic male means that one's sense of childhood is cut short, and the need to be hyper-aware of your surroundings to avoid violence and abuse is frequent."[68] Neurodivergent Black women are also at risk of violence, as autistic writer and advocate Tiffany Hammond explains: "The more I reveal myself, the louder my autism becomes. This means it will be more difficult to keep my behaviors under control and in a world that polices skin like mine the way it does, masking can be a matter of survival as it is a method of hiding."[69]

Although Mewshaw is white, she takes these intersections into account when collaborating with clients on their therapy plans. She told me, "When I'm talking with Black clients, I have to be aware that the way that they move through the world with masking is not going to be the same as my white clients."[70] She doesn't press her own agenda about the "right way" to do therapy onto her clients, especially clients of color who face challenges that white clients will not: "I also always want to respect the ways that they're teaching and discussing masking within their household." For example, she told me, "It's not safe a lot of the time to be a large, Black, autistic man in the world. And so [collaboration] becomes even more relevant when there are intersectionalities at play." But as a white person, Mewshaw will never fully understand the full complexities of being Black in the United States. Ideally, there would be access to Black therapists for all Black children and families. Right now, there is not.

In the face of social pressures to conform to neurotypicality, what, as parents, can we do? We can recognize that the pressures that we feel to make our kids seem more neurotypical are social and institutional and that the norms that teachers enforce aren't set in stone. The same goes for coaches, camp counselors, and others who are supposed to care for our children. We know our kids best, despite the cultural pressure to see outsiders as authority figures. These pressures might also come from our parents (the kids' grandparents) or neighbors. All around us, there are social pressures telling us that our kids need to change. First, we must learn to recognize that these ableist pressures exist in the first place; then, we must recognize that these pressures telling us that our kids must change to meet some neurotypical norm are dead wrong.

For example, a teacher might tell us that it's wrong that our kindergarten child can't tie their shoes. We might feel bad about that, even frustrated or angry. But let's ask: Why *must* a kindergartener, or even a first, second, or third grader, be able to tie their shoes? I'm in my forties, and I still dislike tying shoes. I put elastic laces in every pair of sneakers I buy, and the rest are slip-ons or zip-ups. But when a teacher, an authority figure, told me years ago that my kid's shoes kept coming untied and I needed to *do something about that*, I tried to teach him how to tie them. I tried and tried, and he melted down under all the pressure I put on him. It was a terrible day.

What could I do? I researched all of the wonderful slip-on sneakers they make these days, and we've never bought sneakers with laces again. My kid, the one I traumatized for hours because his teacher shamed me, is fifteen now, and he still gets annoyed by laces. When I look back now at parenting moments I regret, it becomes clear that when I caused my children pain, I was heavily influenced by outside forces telling me that they needed to be something different than they are (and that I was a failure as a parent).

It's our job, as parents, to figure out what matters and what doesn't. Shoelaces? Scratchy fabric? Button-down shirts? They just don't matter. Is it okay that your kid wants to wear headphones to cancel out noise? (I'm wearing mine as I write this, and my kids are wearing theirs in the other room.) Is it okay that your kids interrupt each other and you a lot? Is it okay if they find waiting hard and tend to fidget? Is it okay that they get really frustrated, and I mean really, really frustrated, when things don't come easily at first? Is it okay that they need time alone at family gatherings, even when your family might perceive the behavior as antisocial or rude? Yes. All of these differences are okay, even though our society, and even your friends and family, will pressure and shame you into believing that they are not.

My suggestion is this: Sit down and make a list of conflict points in your house. When do you fight most with your kids? Then ask yourself if these conflicts truly matter. Ask yourself how much you can set aside in order to have a better relationship with your kid and ensure that your kid is less likely to emotionally dysregulate and then melt down. Your kid doesn't need to learn to tough it out or get more resilient. They tough it out every day just being who they are. Instead, they need to learn how to set good boundaries and stand up for themselves and what they need. *That* is what it means to be tough. And we can teach them that. As a bonus, you will have a much better relationship with your kid.

Years ago, when my kids were younger, my family was on vacation in Washington, DC. The four of us—my husband, Eight, Ten, and I—traveled by Metro around town, the train itself as exciting to my sons as the museums and monuments. One time, we exited onto the train platform and the tunnel suddenly grew loud and chaotic because the train across from us let its passengers off at the same time.

My older son, Ten, turned to me, eyes wide: *It's too much.*

I pulled him close and raised his jacket hood, saying, "Cover your ears."

Dipping his chin, he put his hands over his ears, and I kept my arm around him, squeezing him close. Together, we walked to the escalator. I held him as we rode up, and by the time we reached the top, the crowd had dispersed.

He pulled his hands from his ears, dropping his hood. He looked up at me, saying, "Thanks, Mom."

"No problem, buddy," I told him. And it wasn't.

CHAPTER 4

The Medication Double Bind

A double bind is a situation in which a person faces two conflicting demands, usually from some force more powerful than they are. The neurodivergent medication double bind that parents face looks like this. On the one hand, there is immense social pressure for ND kids to conform to social norms, and many people believe these kids should take medication in order to stay in line. On the other hand, there is a societal trend to believe that some (or many) neurodivergences are fake—for example, overdiagnosed or invented by pharmaceutical companies or doctors—and so the medication that parents give kids is unwarranted.

Take ADHD, for example. Ableist norms pressure parents to medicate children who have ADHD so they are less annoying. (I felt this pressure from my kids' schoolteachers.) At the same time, ableism also creates social myths that ADHD is fake, that it doesn't require medication at all, and that Adderall is a drug for fakers and cheaters.

So which is it?

Because of intense social pressure, medication can be the source of many emotions: embarrassment, fear, and shame. But the relationship between a neurodivergent person and their medication is, and should be, a personal one between your family and a doctor that you trust.

UNSOLICITED OPINIONS

It is a hot July, and I'm at a barbecue dinner party with my husband and two boys, ages Eight and Ten. My husband is outside on the patio while I lean against the long counter in the kitchen. A man approaches me with his thick gray hair cropped short and his white skin lined and tanned from time in the outdoors. The man, let's call him Brian, wears athletic sandals and nylon shorts with many pockets. His T-shirt is made of repurposed material, or so the screen printing proclaims. Despite his conventional unconventionality, he seems kind.

"I've been wanting to tell you something all evening," he says. "Do you have a minute?"

Do I? The screen doors to the big wooden house swing open frequently as the dozen or so children dash in and out. Some of those children are mine. Because they are neurodivergent, I feel more pressure to keep a close eye on them than other parents might feel, but from where I'm standing, my kids seem to be all right—happily occupied and safe.

"Sure, I have a minute." I grab a bottle of beer and take a seat on a barstool.

Brian sits at the table next to me. "I have the worst allergies," he says.

This is not the oddest conversation starter I've ever experienced at a dinner party, but then, I went to graduate school for an entire decade. "Really?"

"Don't you?" he asks. "It seems like you do. You've been sniffling a lot."

At this point, I still think Brian is making small talk, albeit odd small talk. "I do have allergies."

Brian nods sagely. "I'd like to tell you about an amazing treatment that my wife and I have used."

I prepare myself for a massively uncomfortable conversation. *He's going to try to sell me something.*

"My wife used to get headaches," Brian says. "But after this treatment"—he goes on to describe a particular type of tea and some other herbal remedy—"her headaches disappeared." He snaps his fingers, his glassy blue eyes bright. "It has to do with inflammation of the brain and the gut."

He goes on, talking more about the gut and the brain, inflammation and tea. I'm now thinking about dessert. Then, his next words hit me like a thunderclap: "And I thought it would help your boys with their problems."

"What?" I'm sure I misheard while eyeing the key lime pie.

"If you stabilized their gut," he says, "it would help your boys with their problems."

He keeps talking, but my brain stopped processing his words after I heard *boys* and *problems*. I set down my beer and walk away.

Outside, I find my husband. Taking his hand, I lead him away from the house and to a far corner of the grassy yard. I try to explain, but I'm sure I'm not making any sense. Words spill out: *allergies* and *guts* and *inflammation* and *our babies* and *that asshole.* I throw my arms around my husband and smush my face against his shoulder and weep. "How could he possibly think it was okay to say those things to me?"

Brian's interaction with me was a type of social policing. After a brief observation of my kids in a semipublic space, he told me that my kids had problems that needed fixing without asking me (or them) if I thought the same. He then took it a step farther, telling me that I should put his dodgy herbs into my children's bodies as though it would be better to experiment on my children with products recommended by a stranger, one who thinks my children are flawed.

If you are not a parent of a ND child, you might wonder whether there is a good way to approach a parent about their kid being ND. While some parents might not mind, in general, you should not walk up to a stranger (or acquaintance) and ask, "Hey, is your kid [insert diagnosis here]?" Why not? For one, many kids don't have diagnoses. Plus, behaviors alone do not equal neurodivergence. Furthermore, neurodivergent kids deserve their privacy, including their medical privacy. I have never shared my children's diagnoses unless required to by schools. If a kid's neurodivergence is important, a parent will tell you. And finally, never, ever give unsolicited advice about how to cure a kid.

As we enter into a discussion on medication, I will begin by saying that if a doctor ever makes you feel the way Brian made me feel, you should take your children and run. (If you are ND and seeking care for yourself, do the same.) As we think about medication for our children, we should avoid making the decision because of outside pressure for our kids to conform to social norms, even though this pressure can be unbelievably heavy. Social pressure to force neurodivergent kids to act "normal," that is, according to neurotypical standards, comes from all angles: our own families, teachers, camp counselors, and strangers at dinner parties. This pressure can be insidious, in the form of social policing with eye rolls and scoffs that make parents feel like they're failing their kids.

Even doctors aren't immune to neurotypical social pressures. A doctor should address the struggles or health issues that interfere with your child's enjoyment of life, not the feelings of others who might wish that your child behaved in a certain way. They should view your child as a whole person, not just a bundle of inconvenient behaviors, taking only those negative behaviors into account. They should treat you like the loving, concerned, attentive parent that you are. Shame should not be at the heart of any doctor's visit or treatment choice. Furthermore, the best doctors involve children in this decision-making, not just parents. They want to get to know children. Finding doctors like this may take persistence, time, and energy. But it is worth it.

Finally, the decision whether to use medication should be based on what will make your kid most happy and able to live a fulfilling life, whatever that looks like for your kid and your family.

MEDICATION SHAMING

At the beginning of the theatrical trailer for Sofia Coppola's satirical film *The Bling Ring* (2013), a mother calls upstairs, "Girls! Time for your Adderall!"[1] The line is both the joke and the punchline, the opening volley of a biopic about drug- and booze-addled high schoolers who robbed movie stars. The scene then cuts to the girls at a nightclub, showing the teens drinking and doing drugs. This opening scene insinuates that Adderall is one of the many drugs the kids abuse, even though it is prescribed by a doctor and dispensed by a parent.

Medication for ADHD faces particularly harsh social judgment. ADHD is a fraught diagnosis, one that is mocked on TV and in films, joked about casually as an insult or metaphor ("I'm so ADD today!"), and vilified as a fake diagnosis chased by wealthy parents seeking special treatment for their kids. When my kids were diagnosed with ADHD in elementary school, the first thing I felt was relief. I knew how to help them now. The second thing I felt was trepidation, because I knew they would face a tsunami of discrimination. Research shows that many people believe either that ADHD is a fake diagnosis or that it is overdiagnosed. But ADHD is a real, painful disability. I see it every day as my kids struggle with it, and I listen to them tell me stories, sometimes in tears, about how hard it is when they can't focus or control their impulses. ADHD is not fake.

The medicines used to treat ADHD are equally vilified. For example, it's harder for me to get a refill for my kid's Adderall than it was for the oxycodone that I used after my recent spine surgeries. There is a societal belief that prescriptions for Adderall and Ritalin are handed out "like candy."

Neurodivergent comedian Hannah Gadsby sums up much of the social stigma against ADHD in their memoir: "ADHD makes a lot of people very, very angry. Attention deficit hyperactive disorder is not an easy thing to explain. And not just because it is especially complex and has a lot of syllables. The real problem is that too many people have been conditioned to believe that ADHD is a nonsense disease that is not so much overdiagnosed but entirely under-existing." They continue, nailing all of the myths that shroud the diagnosis: "A Western medicine scam made up by pharmaceutical companies who wanted to peddle speed but who were too scared to do business with gangs. A fad. An excuse. A handy label given to energetic young boys with shit parents who give them sugar instead of boundaries."[2]

Researchers are aware of this large-scale misbelief about ADHD, attributing much of it to confusion about what ADHD is. Despite the fact that "ADHD is the most extensively studied pediatric mental health disorder," a large part of the public still believes that it is fake.[3] Studies show that "despite overwhelming scientific evidence of the legitimacy of ADHD as a CNS [central nervous system] neurobiological disorder, the general public appears confused about ADHD: is it a medical illness, a psychiatric syndrome, a mental disorder, a behavioral health disorder, a behavioral problem, a motivational problem, or a school-based learning and socialization problem?" This confusion "further feeds the general perception that ADHD is a socially constructed disorder rather than a valid neurobiological disorder. This increases the public's concern that ADHD is overdiagnosed and stimulants are overprescribed."[4]

Stereotypes about what illness is and should be also sow doubts about the reality of ADHD: "The public perceives that children and adults with a medical disorder should look and act sick, whereas many of the core ADHD symptoms are seen in lively, willful, and exuberant persons." Then there is the fear that people with ADHD (called ADHDers) abuse the drugs they are prescribed. But this belief has been proven false by the research, which actually indicates that those for whom it is prescribed often take less than recommended. In short, "the public's fear that ADHD is overdiagnosed and that stimulants are overprescribed is not generally supported by the current scientific research."[5]

Not only is ADHD real, it is also highly stigmatized, and the stigma can have deadly consequences. What is stigma in this context? Put succinctly, stigma is negative stereotyping of neurodiversity based on irrational beliefs, such as fear of negative behavior. In this instance, there is a societal fear that kids with ADHD are faking it to cheat in school or get illegal drugs. The problem is, kids with ADHD can sense this stigma and often avoid asking for help, even when they need it most. (Their parents can sense it too.)

For example, recent research shows that 27 percent of college students have ADHD, although many of them are undiagnosed.[6] (This research has been replicated.) When I share this number in keynote talks, some audience members believe ADHD is overdiagnosed—after all, how could a quarter of college students have ADHD? Impossible. The belief in overdiagnosis increases the stigma felt by ADHDers because it feels like no one believes their struggles. But the same research shows another important statistic. Among college students generally, 5.5 percent attempt suicide.[7] This number is much too high, and, as a longtime college professor, it is heartbreaking to know that so many of my students are suffering. That same research shows that among college students with ADHD, 13.4 percent attempt suicide. Based on these findings, the researchers declared that "students with ADHD present as an at-risk population upon entry into college" and need to be treated as such by school administrators.[8] Changes in environment (such as going to college) combined with lack of support for ADHD traits can lead to depression and suicide attempts. ADHDers in school don't need stigma; they need care and support.

The research about ADHD holds true for many neurodivergences. Common refrains include "everyone has anxiety," "everyone gets sad sometimes," and "everyone's a little autistic." As parents, we can help our children recognize stigmatizing language and decrease its power and also make sure that our children know how to seek help when they need it.

SCHOOLS AND MEDICATION

One place where the pressure to medicate is strongest is at school. When kids don't stay within the narrow path of acceptable social behavior set by a teacher, teachers punish them—and their parents. This is another manifestation of the individual attention fallacy. Some teachers believe the fix for a kid's supposed bad behavior is to pressure parents into medication. My mother encountered this pressure when I was a kid, and I encountered it as a parent when my kids started school.

I interviewed my mother about the first time she and my father put me on Ritalin, which coincided with the first time I was treated for a neurodivergence.[9] I was in the first grade, age six, and my teacher, Mrs. Strickland (really), demanded that I change or else I would be kicked out of school. My mother described the situation to me: "You would get so upset at school. You would get upset if someone knocked over your crayons. You would line them up just so." For the record, a kid lining up their crayons like my mom described to me should have been tested for autism, but back then, girls just couldn't be autistic. Because of my strange behavior, Mrs. Strickland called my mother in for a meeting: "She called you *emotionally disturbed*. She just didn't have the right vocabulary to describe you. But then neither did I. You have to understand, the way I was raised, school was an authority figure. Teachers were an authority figure." Intimidated by the teacher, my parents called a child psychiatrist, who evaluated me and reassured my parents that I was not, in fact, emotionally disturbed. But I seemed to have ADHD.

My parents didn't know what ADHD was. I started school in the early 1980s, and "ADD with hyperactivity" as a diagnosis was first identified by psychiatrists around that same time. It appeared in the third edition of the *Diagnostic and Statistical Manual of Mental Disorders* (*DSM-III*), published in 1980.[10] The doctor's words, even to my well-educated parents, must have seemed mysterious.

My mother said that the doctor "told us about ADHD and a lot of other things we'd never heard about." Even though the doctor was kind and calm, my mom was stressed out by my behavior at the doctor's office: "I remember she had you draw a person on a blackboard in her office. And you drew and drew and drew, so detailed. You even drew the fingernails. The fingernails were really important."

Finally, the psychiatrist offered to have me try Ritalin. Although I was only six, I remember taking Ritalin, and I remember not liking it. The medicine made me anxious and sad. I remember sitting in the cozy brown leather chair in our family room when I came home from school and crying for no reason.

My mom recounted similar memories of my time on the medicine: "You told me that the medicine was making you feel weird. It really suppressed your appetite and that was really stressful to you. You told me, 'I can never eat my lunch. That makes me sad.' You identified that."

Because of my bad reaction to the medicine, my parents took me off of it, and that was the end of my parents' attempt to find a medicine that might help me. When I asked my mom about Mrs. Strickland and her ultimatum, she replied, "We sent you back to school, and it just . . . worked out." I only had a few more months of first grade, my mom told me, and she did everything she could to encourage the teacher to tolerate me in class. She signed me up for weekly social skills therapy with a counselor. Apparently, this intervention was enough to keep my first-grade teacher happy, and I made it through the year.

Decades later, when my own kids started school, I faced similar pressure to change my child to appease a teacher. My younger son was five and starting kindergarten at a private school. Our first school, a public magnet school, had failed to provide adequate services for our older son, Seven. We were, in a word, desperate for a school that could teach our children. Seven was thriving in the classroom of an incredibly patient and kind second-grade teacher. But Five, just starting school, was struggling in his classroom. After sending home note after note, his teacher finally called his father and me in for a meeting. She provided a litany of his terrible behavior. He didn't put his coat away properly, the teacher said. He didn't put his lunch away properly, either. He didn't follow directions at all, she told us. But then things got worse, and he started hiding under his desk. In the meeting, she told my husband and me that in all her years of teaching, she'd never had such a difficult student, and she didn't know what she was going to do with him. She was throwing up her hands. All her efforts had been fruitless. Then she looked at me. Underneath her words, I heard the threat. *Fix him, or else.*

Coincidentally, at the suggestion of a kind speech therapist in our lives, my older son was being evaluated for ADHD by our pediatrician later that week. I was planning to make an appointment for Five as well. So, in my panic during the meeting, I blurted out, "He's seeing someone for ADHD!" My brain, reaching for a lifesaver, thought these words about a diagnosis and possible medication would appease the teacher. And I was right—they did. The teacher nodded gravely, as though she were an integral part of the planning committee deciding my kid's psychiatric treatment and was now giving her approval. Suddenly, my gut sickened. I felt like I had betrayed Five, even though my goal had been to protect him. I still feel that way. Why? Because I allowed myself to be bullied by his teacher and then chose to appease her by sharing his medical information.

Perhaps, later, I would have shared his diagnosis with her, on my terms, to improve his education. But in that panicked moment, on her terms, I folded under her pressure and broke his confidence. Just like my own mother did decades before. Just like countless other desperate parents do. After all, we want teachers to like our children and to take good care of them, and we too fear the stigma that educators and other professionals attach to certain diagnoses, even though they should know better.

Five was evaluated for ADHD by our pediatrician, and sure enough, he was diagnosed along with his brother. But we were lucky. Our doctor was kind and supportive of my children and of neurodiversity. I was also able to figure out that the kindergarten teacher was a bully, and I stood up for my kid after that. It helped that I tentatively mentioned to another parent whose kids had attended the school longer than mine, "I'm not sure my kid likes his teacher." And the other mom scoffed, saying, "What's to like?" Her words were the first crack in the teacher's impenetrable reputation. Teachers can be dictators, and schools are often unable to do much about it given teacher tenure and other perks of seniority. Under this regime, parents often have no choice but to fall in line.

We have also had the wonderful experience of a caring teacher raising the issue of the neurodivergence of a child in order to help and collaborate with us. My older kid's ADHD was first suggested to me by his speech and language pathologist. Before that, we had originally sought the help of an SLP for his dyslexia because his kindergarten teacher recommended it. Then, later, his teacher encouraged us to have him tested for autism, which inspired us to have both kids tested. We're grateful that we had those teachers to help us. Teachers can be a great resource to help you understand your kid's neurodivergences if they have your kid's best interests at heart.

Our quest for diagnoses and medication was relatively easy. During the process, the pediatrician and I discussed diagnoses with my kids. We talked to them about how they were feeling. We asked them if they wanted to try medicine to help them focus. I named it "focus medicine" (and we still call Adderall that today, even though they know its actual name now). Later, as their diagnoses became more complex, we found a wonderful psychiatrist. He always talks directly to the kids, not just with us parents. He has helped the kids understand their own bodies and brains (they're one thing!), teaching them how to tell whether the medicine is helping and to understand the side effects to look out for. When the doctor raised the dose of a medicine and my kid didn't like it, the doctor lowered it. There was dialogue and education so that my children were able to participate in their own care, which is a crucial lifelong skill for neurodivergent people.

When I was a kid, given time and trial, we might have found a medicine that would have helped me. But for that to have happened, my parents and I would have needed an accurate diagnosis to begin with and ongoing support for medication. I'm lucky that my mother convinced the school to let me stay despite dropping the medicine. Her explanation, *it just . . . worked out*, is not one that every parent encounters. Sometimes schools do not give ND kids the leeway they deserve even when parents try their best with medication for their child.

THE IMPATIENCE OF SCHOOLS

One challenge parents and kids face with medicine is that finding the right medicine and dose can take some time. Along the way, things can be rocky. For example, one medicine might make a kid sleepy in school or have a paradoxical reaction—for example, making a behavior worse than it was before. But in my experience, and in the experience of parents I interviewed, many schools don't have patience for this important time in a kid's life. They want a quick fix.

I interviewed Anastasia, a white, cisgender mother of two adopted ND kids, about her experiences with school and medicine.[11] Her stories show how much intolerance schools can have for ND kids trying to find the right medicine (alongside other therapies). Anastasia has anxiety, and although she was never formally diagnosed, she suspects she is AuDHD (autistic and ADHD). She is trained as an architect and has taught design at the university level for three years. She recently graduated with a degree in project management and will be applying for jobs in higher education administration. She says her experience in teaching has given her a new perspective on how education works, and doesn't work, for ND students. Her older child ("Older") is eleven and has ADHD, autism, and anxiety. They are also trans and use the pronouns they/them.

Although her family now lives in the Northeast, for a long while, they lived in the South for work. There, they struggled to find adequate schooling for Older, who is twice exceptional ("2E"), which means they are both gifted and in need of support at school. The family moved to a larger city an hour away so that Older could attend a unique private school that specialized in children like Older. The school promised that Older would fit in nicely in the school community. At this time, Older was eight years old.

After a few months, things seemed fine. Then one day in the fall, Anastasia received a phone call from the school social worker, one that was familiar to her after receiving many similar ones from other schools in the past: "She said, 'We're concerned about safety.' It's a big buzzword, safety. And as soon as I hear that, I say, *Oh, shit, here we go again*, because as soon as they say it's an issue with safety, you know that they're starting to open the door to ask you to leave, and that's true across the board and has been always so." Anastasia's fear came true: "Then the next thing I know I get a call . . . from the principal. She told me that [Older] had sworn at the teacher and that wasn't acceptable to them and that they wanted [Older] to leave."

When I asked her how she felt about the swift expulsion of eight-year-old Older from school, she told me she felt "angry" and "pissed" because "they weren't even willing to have a conversation about it." In fact, the main issue that bothered Anastasia was medication: "They knew we were trying different medications because this was the first time we've seen a psychiatrist. And I was like, obviously this medication isn't working. We're trying different ones, like we're in the process of trying different things."

But despite her explanations and pleas, the school "didn't have any interest in it." As much as Anastasia was trying to find the right medicine for her kid so that they could be safe, happy, and successful, the school didn't give her family time to work through the process. She pointed out that they could have had Older sit out the rest of that semester and come back in January, but they didn't give them that option. Although public schools have more red tape when it comes to expelling a child, they can still suspend your child without notice. (I've been there.) If you are the parent of a ND kid, I recommend that you research the school punishments in your state and ways to appeal them.

INVOLVING YOUR KID IN MEDICATION DECISIONS

The decision to use medication can and should be made with the goals of your child and your family in mind. Ideally, you make this decision with your child. When my kids first started taking medicine for their neurodivergences, we collaborated on the decision; they understood far more than I expected them to—and I already expected a lot because they're awesome. Other parents have had similar positive experiences with medication when they take a collaborative approach free from the pressure to force their kid inside the lines of "normal."

To learn more about the decision to choose medication, I interviewed Sophia, a straight, white, cisgender woman whose son is AuDHD.[12] She told me, "We've been purposeful about helping him to develop a positive neurodivergent identity." That purposeful stance has translated to how they, as a family, handle his medicine. When I asked Sophia about her experience with medication for her kid, she told me that he takes Ritalin (the brand name for methylphenidate), which is a nervous system stimulant commonly used to treat ADHD. She said that her son is very open about taking the medicine and understands how it affects his body. He knows not to drink caffeine when he's taken it because there are negative interactions. When I asked her about how the medicine has worked, she said, "It would not be exaggerating to say it's been a game changer for him."

In our interview, she explained to me the process for coming to the decision to try medicine with her son, which was collaborative: "When we started the medication for my son, I asked him, 'Is this something you want to try? Here's what it might do. Here's how it might help.' And he was actually really excited and happy to try it, which let me know as a parent, 'Oh, this must have been really stressful for him, feeling this lack of being able to focus, if he is so excited to try something that might help.'" I asked her about how the medicine has helped him, and she explained, "It does exactly what it's supposed to do for him." She explained, "I know it doesn't work for everybody the same way. And people need to talk to their doctors about what will work." But she says that for her son, Ritalin has improved his quality of life in all environments; for example, "when he is going out into public to do something that he wants to do, that he wants to enjoy, but he's incapable of controlling the frenetic movements, the energy, and his mind enough to enjoy it, [the medicine] allows him not only to focus on academics but to carry on conversations with people and to enjoy things that he wants to enjoy."

She told me a story about a collaborative conversation she had with her son after he first started his medicine to help him understand how it is supposed to work, a great model for how to communicate to a kid about medicine and help them understand:

> The first day he tried it was during the virtual school year [during COVID-19]. He took the first pill. He wanted me to film him taking it. As in, "Here I am trying my new brain medicine," which is what we called it at first before we explained, "This is actually called Ritalin." It was just brain medicine. He wanted me to film this momentous occasion for him, and so he swallowed it. He was happy.
>
> And then he went to his classes. In his math class, he got a problem wrong. . . . And [the teacher] explained how to do the problem and where he went wrong. He listened. He was like, "Oh, okay." After we turned off the monitor from the virtual class, he was very upset. He said, "The pill didn't work. I got that math problem wrong."
>
> I realized we had to have a talk about what you can expect from this pill. I explained that it's not a magic pill. "That doesn't mean that you're never going to get a math problem wrong. But did you notice how, after you got the problem wrong, when the teacher was explaining it to you, you were really listening? And you understood the explanation?" And he said, "Yeah." And I said, "That's what the pill was helping you to do."

As Sophia's story shows, even for a kid in elementary school (as her son was when he started Ritalin), consent and collaboration are not only possible but also key to an empowering relationship between a kid and their medicine. Ensuring that our kids understand how the medicine works not only ensures that they can live better lives but also keeps them safe because they can tell us when it makes them feel poorly or is not working like it is supposed to. It also teaches kids bodily autonomy and boundaries because they have a say about what happens to their bodies.

MEDICINE IS (ONLY) FOR YOUR KIDS, NOT TO PLEASE ADULTS

My kids and I take medicine for our neurodivergences, and we wouldn't have it any other way. But the double bind means that there are those who would foist medicine (be it weird tea or Adderall) upon us and those who tell us that the drugs we take are poison. No matter what we do, someone has an opinion, and they believe it is their right to share it. Among people I'm on speaking terms with and who know about my neurodivergences, some still believe they have the right to voice an unsolicited opinion. Some think that medication will somehow make my health worse. They say it will crush my creative spirit. It will cause horrible side effects. It will harm my unborn (likely never-to-be-born) third or fourth children—a moot point now because I recently had a hysterectomy. They say it's addictive. That it's morally wrong.

I have bipolar disorder (among other things), and I take medication for it. Approximately 4.4 percent of people in the United States have bipolar disorder, and studies show that most people in the United States say they are afraid of people with bipolar disorder.[13] Furthermore, bipolar disorder is a deadly illness, with approximately 20 percent of people who have it dying by suicide.[14] Medication for me is, without exaggeration, a lifesaver. I've been on psychiatric medication since I was twenty-one years old. In all those years, I've encountered few side effects, and it has let me live a life that I love. And yet the criticism doesn't stop.

In our society, people feel entitled to share uninformed opinions about medicine and neurodivergent people—or really anything at all about us. Our bodies and lives are open for public discussion. This privilege stems from ableism. If neurodiversity were embraced by our society, then the privacy of neurodivergent people, including children, would be treated with respect. When discussion centers ND kids, opinions blow in like a hurricane. In the name of "doing what's best for kids," everyone seems to have an opinion.

If you are faced with outsiders trying to give you advice, you have some choices. You can reflect their words back to them. If someone says, "I would never medicate my child," you can say, "I'm happy to hear you would make a different choice for your child." You can question the source of their opinion: "Have you been researching this for some time? Tell me about it." You can also take a stronger approach: "Are you meaning to give me unsolicited medical advice that contradicts our doctor?"

As parents, when we're forced to listen to these opinions, either in the public sphere or from family, friends, or teachers, doubts about our own decisions can slip in. Are we doing the right thing? It can be really hard to push those voices aside and choose a path that works best for our families, but we must. Even well-intentioned opinions don't take lived experiences into account.

We must also surround ourselves with professionals we trust, such as doctors, mental health professionals, education specialists, and others who listen not only to us but also to our children, who take their time and don't rush us out of the room or just to immediate, handy diagnoses. We must find therapists who help our children embrace who they are instead of squeezing them into a box of neurotypical conformity. All professionals we work with must be willing to collaborate with us rather than boss us and our kids around. Finding help like this is hard. Please don't give up.

My own kids, now thirteen and fifteen, take medicine for their neurodivergences, and, according to them, their lives are better because of it. Medicine in our house is a collaborative affair. My kids can tell how their medicine affects them, just like six-year-old me could tell that my medicine was making me feel bad. We talk about their medicine constantly, and always have, and I respect their opinions, as does their psychiatrist, whom they meet with privately and who respects their decisions. They understand what they're taking and what it's for. They know when it is and isn't working right, and they tell me.

Most importantly, I'm not looking for a cure—not for them and not for me. No treatment of any kind is meant to make my kids conform to the needs of an inflexible teacher or an inflexible world or some jerk at a party. Their chosen treatment is not for anyone but them. It is a tool to help them enjoy their lives to the fullest.

CHAPTER 5

School Accommodations

One of my earliest and best memories from elementary school is this: We were all sitting on the floor around our teacher in the gifted education classroom, where we spent a few hours every week. She held a black crayon and a sketch pad in her hand. With a few strokes of that crayon, she drew a tree that looked so lifelike I had to sit on my hands to keep from touching the paper. Granted, I sat on my hands a lot back then because I had impulse-control issues and my regular teacher insisted I sit on my hands a lot.

Then the teacher handed all of us a crayon and an oversized piece of paper and taught us about shadows, branches, and how to imagine what trees really looked like. She showed us how to draw what we saw, not what we were told to see. No more cotton candy trees for us. She'd raised our expectations for ourselves.

She raised our expectations for ourselves across the board—not just in art. In her class, I read my first chapter book. I was just starting first grade, and no one had ever given me a chapter book before. But she had no doubt that we could do it. After giving us each a copy and telling us to go home and read it, she told us to underline the words we didn't know and to look them up in a dictionary. I read the book in one weekend, and there were lots of words I had to underline.

For decades after, I wrote the words I didn't know inside the back covers of books I read, until those lists got shorter and shorter and then disappeared altogether. Pulling old books off my bookshelves today, my copies of Robin McKinley or Cynthia Voigt, of *From the Mixed-Up Files of Mrs. Basil E. Frankweiler* or *A Wrinkle in Time*, I flip open the back covers and see how this gifted education teacher taught me how to challenge myself and hold myself accountable when no one else would.

What would my life have been like without her? How would I have seen the trees? How would I have encountered words? How would I have perceived myself when my first-grade teacher told me, indirectly, that I didn't even belong in school?

Part of me has always wondered: Given how tenuous my situation was in my elementary school, how did I get into the gifted program in the first place?

A few years back, a friend shared that her son was selected for the gifted program in our local public schools "even though his writing looks like a monkey's." Her kid is a few years older than mine, and I remember thinking, with an aching heart, two different things: My kids would benefit so much from the special challenges and creative projects that kids get to do in the gifted program. And my kids will never, ever be accepted into any school's gifted program, no matter what their test scores say, because their grades do not reflect their intellectual potential. In the end, it turned out that the problem was not one of grades or scores but of logistics. When it comes to schools, logistics are often the thing that matters most.

THE FEAR OF ASKING FOR TOO MUCH

First thing in the morning on a day in early April of 2019, I am about to send an email to the school psychologist on behalf of my fourth grader, Nine. I have just received a bulk-mail email from the school system letting us know that, now that the testing for the gifted program has passed, notices of acceptances will come out in a month or two. I think, *When was the testing? And why did no one tell me about the gifted program before?*

Earlier that year, we enrolled Seven and Nine in the local public school. The year before that, we homeschooled them. The year before that, they attended a private school that we hoped would be a good fit because of the smaller class sizes and the school's ability to customize education for kids like mine—kids who are exceptionally bright and also have exceptional needs. The private school failed us, hence the homeschooling.

Now I'm sitting in front of my laptop, my work forgotten as my head spins with desperate plans and strategies to help my kids, the constant plight of a parent of ND kids in a world that pushes them to the margins. I decide to forward the gifted program email to the school psychologist. I like her a lot and believe she's on my kids' side, wanting what's best for them. Later, she would be the one who supported in-school testing for my older son for autism. And when the school said they would not recommend testing my younger son, she encouraged me to seek it privately so he could also get the school services he needed.

But before I can send the email, I'm struck by self-doubt. The week before, I met with the school psychologist and the rest of the exceptional children (EC) team to finalize the details of my children's individualized education programs (IEPs) and 504 plans for their ADHD and language-acquisition struggles. The reason I missed the gifted deadline, I think, is because I've spent the past months working with the school on disability accommodations for my kids. Then I wonder whether, in the eyes of the school, if my kids need accommodations, then they would not need gifted education.

My kids' test scores with psychologists reveal that they are "gifted." They are what is called "twice exceptional," or 2E, just like I was, which means they have exceptional intellectual gifts and exceptional educational needs. Like many 2E kids, my kids' grades don't reflect their raw abilities—not yet. That's what the accommodations are for. But, just like other gifted students, my kids need what they would get in the gifted program: the intellectual and creative challenges that will keep them interested in school. I want them to love school instead of fretting about it or getting bored and hating it. I believe that they need school in order to meet other kids like them. They need it to reach their potential. They also need it to be happy, which is my number one priority.

But as I fret, I wonder why it is that every time I ask for what my kids need to reach their full potential, I fear I am asking for too much? Why do I feel as though I'm only allowed to request that one exceptionality be accommodated? I don't know why it is so hard to see that a kid can be both disabled and gifted. I'm describing the challenge that every parent of a 2E kid faces. We are begging the world, "Please see my kid as more than his challenges. Please see his gifts as well." I go so far as to argue that this is the challenge every parent of *every* ND kid faces, even those without the 2E label. Some kids' gifts are hidden from society by a kid's high support needs; those needs are often all anyone will see.

As I compose the email to the psychologist, I frame it with a question, rather than a statement of fact—"Is the gifted program something that my kids might be eligible for?"—and send it. I ask myself, *If I don't advocate for my kids, then who will?* Still, a part of me wonders if I'm asking too much. I'm afraid of becoming one of *those moms* who bullies the school into making way for my kids.

Now, in retrospect, I don't have qualms about being one of those moms. Advocating for your kid is not bullying. All these years later, I see that I was the one who was bullied by multiple school administrations that did not want to see ND students as individuals but rather shoved them into cookie-cutter programs that were easier for them to implement and that utterly failed my children. I interviewed many parents for this book, and not one of them has been satisfied with the accommodations schools provide. Some, like me, have had to pay thousands of dollars for private testing. Another had to hire a lawyer to get a proper IEP. More than one opted out of conventional schooling altogether and homeschooled instead—with the funding for disability students that the state provides if you know how to jump through the hoops. What I learned from all of this research is this: Don't give up. You are your child's best advocate.

A few weeks after I emailed the school psychologist, my son brings me a sealed envelope from his backpack. "This had your name on it, Mom," he tells me, then runs from my office to do his homework in the kitchen. The return name on the brown manila envelope is the gifted director at our school.

I open it and extract two sheets of paper, each with one of my son's names at the top. Each document expresses that my child has been designated for the gifted program based on testing I've already submitted for their IEPs—no new testing is required. The letters are impersonal form letters, with names and numbers handwritten into empty places, but the underlying message is clear: My email worked.

Leaning back in my chair, I think about the many invisible struggles I've had to face while sitting here at my desk. I think about how that's what it means to be a parent of any child, not just children like mine or like I was. You have doubts, and you feel guilt, but you push it all aside and hope you're doing the right thing.

Thirty years ago, my mom had doubts about me. When I was in first grade and starting the gifted program, I was nearly kicked out of school by my regular classroom teacher because of my behavior. I had trouble sitting still, sitting in rows, sitting quietly, staying interested in things that I already knew or that bored me, waiting quietly while doing nothing, and remembering complex directions. There were so many things about this teacher's classroom that made me miserable.

I remember a change happening in the middle of the school year. I don't know whose idea it was, but I'm grateful. After I finished my classwork, I no longer had to sit and do nothing. I was allowed to sit on the floor and write stories. The blank storybooks were made of oversized newsprint, with lines on the bottom and white space on the top for drawing, side-stapled like a real book. I was allowed to use as many of the books as I wanted. So whenever I had extra time, I took out a storybook and wrote and drew, letting my imagination loose. I wrote complex stories with dialogue and talking animals. I wrote stories that spanned multiple storybooks, each one a chapter. And the trees I drew were beautiful.

Every student should have the chance to learn in a way that encourages their imagination and challenges their mind. But most children don't have that kind of schooling. For ND kids, school can become a nightmare of overstimulation combined with rigid and complex rules paired with confusing punishments and academic failures. The laws that require accommodations for ND and other disabled kids are supposed to protect against punishments and failures that arise on the basis of their disabilities. The first thing we must do as parents is learn as much as we can about these rules. I didn't learn enough early enough, and I know I'm not alone. The second thing we must do is figure out what the best learning situation is for our children based on our own family's resources. The best learning situation for a ND kid might not look like "normal" school at all. But we should not be surprised that kids who live outside social norms frequently do not take to a school system that is highly normed.

IEPS, 504S, AND ACCOMMODATIONS

This chapter is not meant to be an accommodations guidebook for parents with ND kids in school. There are outstanding resources out there that cover the laws and guide you through the process. Here, I present a basic overview of the rules and provide resources so that you can dive deeper into the process in your own school district. More importantly, this book provides stories from parents who have faced challenges in order to give you perspectives on how you can approach schooling for your child.

Accommodations for ND and other disabled kids in public schools are handled by IEPs and 504 plans. They are different, although the differences are confusing. The procedures for getting these plans in the first place are also confusing. Here is a brief overview of the differences.

Individual education programs are governed by IDEA, the Individuals with Disabilities Education Act of 2004.[1] For a ND student to qualify for an IEP, they must be enrolled in a publicly funded school, meet criteria for one or more of the fourteen disabling conditions in IDEA (following), and have a disability that adversely affects their educational performance and requires specially designed instruction. Private schools that receive no federal funding are not required to provide IEPs. For example, for one year, my kids attended a Catholic school, and the school did not provide IEPs or accommodations under IDEA. They did provide some reading support for my older son, but otherwise, they failed to support my kids' education. But unlike at a public school, I had no recourse for these failures.

Various laws provide the specific fourteen disability categories that can qualify a student under IDEA: (1) autism, (2) deaf-blindness, (3) deafness, (4) emotional disturbance, (5) hearing impairment, (6) intellectual disability, (7) multiple disabilities, (8) orthopedic impairment, (9) other health impairment (OHI), (10) specific learning disability (SLD), (11) speech or language impairment (SLI), (12) traumatic brain injury (TBI), (13) visual impairment (including blindness), and (14) developmental delay.[2]

But the mere diagnosis is not enough to qualify a student for an IEP. The disability must also adversely affect the student's performance in school. The "adversely affect" standard is subjective, to say the least. During one of my school meetings, I pointed out that my intellectually gifted autistic child was only managing a C average. I told the committee that these grades were well below his academic potential, and in response, the committee told me that the school's job is only to ensure that my kid received *an adequate education, not to reach his potential.* That was the day I lost faith in the accommodations process. What does "adversely affect" mean if not this? If the school only sees my child's deficits and not his gifts, then what is the point?

Although a school is permitted to do more for a child if they choose, IDEA only requires a "free appropriate public education" and no more.[3] A US Supreme Court opinion laid down the law in 1982 when they overturned a lower court decision in favor of a deaf student. The lower court originally held in favor of the student: "Because of this disparity between the child's achievement and her potential, the court held that she was not receiving a 'free appropriate public education,' which the court defined as 'an opportunity to achieve [her] full potential commensurate with the opportunity provided to other children.'" In overturning the lower court, the Supreme Court gave a different definition of a "free appropriate public education." They held that IDEA "does not require a State to maximize the potential of each handicapped child commensurate with the opportunity provided nonhandicapped children."[4] IDEA just gets our kids through the door, nothing more.

But some laws do protect ND families. For example, federal law says that "parents have a right to request an 'independent educational evaluation' (IEE) at public expense if they disagree with the school district's evaluation of their child."[5] Thus, in that meeting, I could have pushed harder to have my younger son evaluated for autism, paid for by the school system. You can too. Federal law also states, "A parent may also provide outside evaluations of the child to the school district in order to allow the IEP Team to consider that information when it is making determinations regarding needed evaluations, eligibility, IEP services and placements, and manifestation determinations for the child."[6] When my older son was in first grade, I had him evaluated by an external speech and language pathologist, which revealed his severe dyslexia. When I shared her evaluation with the school, the administrators ignored it because, they told me, the testing had to be done by the school in order to be valid. This statement was plainly false, but I didn't know it then. I also could have insisted that they do the testing themselves, but I didn't. I now know I could have pointed to this law, and I could also have requested testing by the school, which they would have had to provide based on his own teacher's recommendations.

But I didn't advocate strongly enough because I didn't know how. Instead, he received minimal support, and I paid for a private SLP.

At an IEP meeting, the law requires the attendance of one of the child's teachers, one EC teacher, an administrator who can implement the IEP, and a psychologist or similar who can "interpret the instructional implications of evaluation results," which is sometimes a school psychologist. But some schools or districts don't have all of these personnel, so the meeting won't have them. As parents, you are also entitled to attend (and should), and many parents don't know that they may bring a support person with them. This person can be anyone: a friend, an advocate, or a lawyer. Education advocates are experts in school accommodations who offer advice and attend meetings to assist parents in getting the best accommodations for their children.

IEPs have two main parts: "goals" and "services."[7] Goals refers to the learning goals that the school will set for the student and that the teachers will measure to see if they have been met. Services "help children benefit from special education by providing extra support in needed areas. Examples: speech, occupational or physical therapy, therapeutic recreation, interpretation services, school health and social work services."[8] The school provides services, but it also must quantify improvement based on goals.

A ND child who does not qualify for education accommodations might qualify for a 504 plan. Section 504 plans were created under Section 504 of the Rehabilitation Act of 1973,[9] developed for students who have a disability but do not require special education services.[10] Section 504 "provides civil rights protections to all individuals with disabilities in programs that receive federal funding, which includes public schools."[11] The

Rehabilitation Act "provides protection from discrimination based upon a child's disability, if that disability substantially limits a major life activity, such as talking, walking or learning. Any facility that receives federal assistance is covered by this civil rights law."[12] In short, if a school is excluding a student from any activity, educational or extracurricular, due to disability, a 504 plan ensures that the school provides accommodations and supports to the student so that they can participate.[13]

But these bare facts don't tell the emotional story of the IEP/504 process. The process can be emotionally draining, expensive, and frustrating.[14] Even after you have a plan in place at the administrative level, teachers do not always follow it, which requires more effort on your part to ensure that the teachers are providing the services your child needs. For these reasons, I strongly recommend parents educate themselves about the IEP/504 process, and the services available in their school systems, at least a full year before their kid ever starts school. You might need to do certain testing, for example, and the waitlist for the testing might be six months. You might want to get on the waitlist for a magnet school if there is one available that will better support your child. You might want to hire an advocate to assist you, and the one you want may get booked up fast. Start early.

To learn more about the IEP and 504 process, I interviewed Anthony, a fourth-generation Chinese American originally from Texas who now lives in the southeastern United States.[15] He is a cisgender man and a divorced single father of one child, a son, now aged fourteen, of whom he has majority joint custody. His son was diagnosed with autism at age two and a half and with ADHD around age nine. Anthony himself does not have a formal diagnosis, but he suspects he might be neurodivergent.

Anthony told me how, at the first few school meetings, things did not go well. Although Anthony requested modifications to his son's IEP, school administrators were not receptive. He called the process "mechanistic" and inflexible, telling me, "They seem to have fairly set ideas as to what goals were measurable. And what they could keep data on always baffled me. Especially his general education teachers who are supposed to keep data on this and also be teaching the other twenty-eight students." He's referring to the "goals" portion of the IEP, which states things like "student will be able to do [goal] within 3 months." But Anthony is skeptical of the goals process. He told me, "There have only been a couple of occasions where they [the teachers] have come to the meeting with detailed enough data to make me confident that they were even adhering to the goals or tracking them." He told me that he felt "puzzled," wondering, "Why is everything being framed in terms of goals rather than services?" In other words, Anthony feels like the intense focus that schools put on the goals portion of the IEP overshadows the more important services portion, when the two are supposed to be treated equally.

Early in his son's educational career, Anthony felt like the IEP process was not going well, so he brought education advocates to meetings on three separate occasions. The experience with advocates was a good one, and he learned a lot from them: "Due to the presence of the advocates, we got better results. But it was good to learn from them. You know, how they raise issues in the meetings, and the kind of the scope of issues that could be raised." Many parents do not understand the options that they have at a meeting, and for Anthony, an advocate was able to show him the breadth of options for goals and services he could request for his son. Anthony told me, however, that because he brought an advocate, the school brought their attorney to meetings. In my experience with IEP meetings (two kids, many years), I have never seen an attorney in a meeting, and I *am* an attorney. So I was shocked to hear about an attorney being present, and this may not be the case at every school. At a meeting where parents are already outnumbered and on the defensive, the thought of the school having a lawyer present feels intimidating. When I asked Anthony what the school's lawyer did, he told me, "I don't remember that the lawyer said anything. I think they just brought them on to observe, or maybe whisper things in their ears."

Anthony also told me that he always records the IEP meetings, which I think is a great idea and one I wish I had adopted. But he said that whenever he places his recorder on the table, the school then places theirs. So when you record your meetings, and I strongly suggest you do so, be prepared for the school to record as well.

FINDING A SCHOOL ADVOCATE

To learn more about finding an advocate for IEP and 504 meetings, I interviewed child psychologist Emily King, a former school psychologist who is an expert in IEP/504 settings.[16] She provides helpful advice to families who want better guidance through the process. When I was going through the process, if I had known there were advocates, I would have used one.

What does an advocate do? King explained to me that "advocates review evaluations [e.g., psychological-education testing] with families, help them understand the process and their rights, sometimes help them draft emails to school staff, and can attend meetings with parents." King told me that years ago, most advocates used to be lawyers, which had a negative effect on the process: "When I was a school psychologist fifteen years ago, most of the advocates I met were lawyers. But I do recall that if a family brought a lawyer to a meeting, then the school district brought a lawyer to the meeting and tension was always higher and the meeting longer when lawyers were involved. Sometimes this was necessary, but sometimes it wasn't."

Things have changed, King explained to me: "Special education services advocates I refer to now are not lawyers but have collaborative relationships with school administrators that are helpful when making tough decisions in meetings. Advocates in my area are private businesses, and I know of one that is set up as a nonprofit." So how can parents find advocates? King said, "They use word of mouth or an internet search to find them. Therapists like myself or psychologists doing private testing usually refer families to advocates if the case is complex, if we hear something that doesn't sound like the child is getting what they need at school, or if the parent is really new to the process and needs some hand-holding throughout all the meetings and paperwork. It's a lot of new terminology!"

King provided some "red flags" to look out for when seeking an advocate: "In my opinion, an adversarial advocate who is going to 'fight' for your child and could be argumentative is a red flag. In my experience, this positioning shuts down collaboration and is not helpful for the child, makes meetings longer, and doesn't lead to flexibility with tough decisions."

I don't know what would have happened if we'd had an advocate on our side during the myriad IEP/504 processes our family experienced. I know that the process would have been easier and that we would have gotten better outcomes. Would my kids have stayed in conventional school? I don't know. But they would no doubt have had a better shot.

RACE AND NEGLECT IN PUBLIC SCHOOLS

The barriers to effective IEP/504 accommodations particularly affect poor people and people of color. To learn more about this disparity, I interviewed Cameron, a Black woman and a native North Carolinian.[17] She has an MBA and worked for years in New York City in corporate consulting. She has three children, and her youngest, a six-year-old boy, is autistic. In late 2019, when her youngest was nearly three years old, she and her husband and kids moved back home to North Carolina to be near her family.

Cameron was very disappointed by the dramatic differences between the public-funded support that her son received in New York and the lack of support North Carolina provided. Every state handles public services differently. For example, New York and New Jersey are particularly well known for their services for ND kids. Cameron explained, "I went from having, I would say, platinum-tier services for my child that were provided, regardless of income, in New York, to having literally nothing." When she discovered the services that North Carolina did provide, she found them to be financially out of reach for most families. Either you had to be extremely poor or wealthy like her own family: "What about those people who are working class and in the middle?" Discussing the cost of services, she said, "It wasn't much, but it wasn't insignificant. But there are people who really have to make the choice as to whether to pay $50 a month for this, or I get my kid service for that." The services were disappointing, too. They were, as she put it, "cookie cutter, meant to solve for the gaps in teaching proficiency and not the reality of what these children face."

Cameron, who has done advocacy work in the area of education and ND children, explained how the lack of access to

services and the poor-quality services all around dispropor-
tionately affect Black and Hispanic children: "These [neurodi-
vergent] children end up being pushed into general classrooms because they're not the most severe [i.e., the highest
support needs]. And then they end up becoming behavioral
problems, especially children of color." When schools label
these ND children of color as behavior problems, Cameron
points out, an avalanche of negative events occur: "They are
stigmatized. They may end up in a special needs class anyway
because they don't get the support and attention they need in
a general class. It just leads to a whole cascade of things, so
that by middle school, you have a child that never got the support they need." What about the adults who were supposed to
help these children? The parents, the schools? "The parents
don't necessarily know what to do. The school sees them [the
kids] in a certain way, and now they're hitting puberty, and
they have a whole lot of behaviors that were never addressed
that become problematic." The consequences, Cameron told
me, are tragic: "This is one of the things that might even be a
pipeline to prison for a lot of poor and minority children. That's
the double whammy."

Cameron's observations are backed up by research. In the
context of autism, children from racial minority and under-
served populations experience longer delays in diagnosis than
white children.[18] For example, the average age of diagnosis for
Black children was 65 months compared to a nationwide average of 49 months. When they are older, Black disabled/neuro-
divergent children are more likely to be punished in school
and to have law enforcement called on them by school.[19] In
general, school punishments are more frequently doled out to
students of color. Low-income students and students of color
who are also disabled/neurodivergent face discrimination by

school staff and teachers, with even more frequent punishments coming their way because of the intersection of ableism and racism.[20]

Although Cameron has been very active in the IEP/504 process with her son, she told me that the schools make it easy for parents, especially poor and overworked parents of color, to be more passive: "As an African American parent, it's even more frustrating to see the gaps that truly exist within my community, and some of that self-imposed. We've got parents who are really disengaged." But, she points out, this disengagement is encouraged by schools themselves: "The way the public schools are structured, it makes it easier to disengage. You know the bus will pick them up. You don't have to worry about that. The lunch is crappy, but they'll eat." Schools, then, present a way for overworked parents of color to allow their ND children to be cared for, just not, as Cameron explains, well enough: "So they pacify the parent. And then you have working-class parents who, God bless them! They just don't have a certain level of education to know what red flags to look for." In the end, Cameron believes our education system in the United States, especially in North Carolina, is failing all Black children, ND Black children in particular.

After moving back to North Carolina, Cameron made the tough decision to send her own children to private school (and also private camps) after trying the public options. She told me, "From a Black standpoint, yes, you want your children to be comfortable around Black people of all types. And I want them to be around other Black people." But, after too many experiences finding her ND child abandoned in a corner or otherwise neglected, she felt like her kids were not safe in public schools and camps, telling me, "I wouldn't put my child in a car with no brakes."

TWICE EXCEPTIONAL

Cameron's autistic son, like my own children, is "twice exceptional." Cameron told me that her son, by three years old, "knew his sight words. He could count to 100. He knew his colors." How did he learn these things? "That was us homeschooling. He wasn't talking much, but when you asked him, he could name things. By the time he was four, he had memorized the multiplication table." Although he needed support services in school, he also needed intellectual challenges. But Cameron didn't have faith that schools would provide these challenges. My own experience as a 2E parent bears this out.

Experts have loosely divided 2E students into three categories:[21]

- Students whom schools have identified as gifted but who then struggle in school because their disabilities aren't supported. Often these students are labeled as "underachievers." Because their disabilities remain unidentified, "as school becomes more challenging, their academic difficulties may increase to the point where they are falling sufficiently behind peers that someone finally suspects a disability."

- Students who have disabilities that are so severe that schools recognize them, but schools fail to recognize their intellectual gifts. Far more frequently than we imagine, these students' "potential remains unrecognized," and "it never becomes a cause for concern or the focus of their instructional program."

- Students whose strengths and struggles mask one another. These students "sit in general classrooms, ineligible for services provided for students who are gifted or have learning disabilities and are considered to have average abilities." They perform at grade level and are not "a priority for schools on tight budgets."

This research tracks with the anecdotal research I have conducted. For example, as Anthony told me, "I was very concerned that the service provision would be affected by [my son's] talents masking his struggles and vice versa."[22] This talents/struggles conflict was one of the reasons that getting an effective IEP was so difficult for Anthony's son.

As researchers have noted as a common occurrence with 2E kids who lack adequate support, Anthony's son's performance trended downward as the material grew more difficult, especially in reading, where he has more struggles. In his elementary school years, Anthony's son won spelling bees. But as he progressed through middle school, Anthony told me, his language arts grades trended downward: "He actually had very high [abilities] in reading. In spelling, he's so fastidious. In the formal writing, at the same time, his writing is not fluent. He'll do the absolute minimum to answer the questions. And his ability to abstract or get the main ideas [aren't strong]. . . . So he had off-the-charts reading scores, and those have drifted downward, in everything but math."

And yet, Anthony told me that if he were to seek an IEP for his son today, he doesn't believe his son would be eligible for one because his son is performing too well in school to meet the criteria. Although his reading scores have fallen, he's not doing poorly enough—in the eyes of the school system—to warrant the support: "His grades are good enough that if we were applying for eligibility now, I'm not sure he would [get an IEP]. We might have a struggle getting it because he's done well in school.

But pretty clearly he does have special support needs in the curriculum as well as for behavior."

When my older son was eight, he encountered a teacher who labeled him an underachiever. In third grade, his teacher tormented him because he couldn't replicate the perfect handwriting she demanded for every assignment. She refused to believe that he needed accommodations for dysgraphia (struggles with handwriting), which often accompanies his other neurodivergences. We had given her an IEP that told her to essentially ignore his poor handwriting, but she did not. I had the testing psychologist write a letter directly to her explaining my son's disability, and she ignored it. She believed that he simply needed to work harder and lovely handwriting would manifest. And since, in her eyes, he wasn't trying hard enough, she frequently punished him.

For example, Eight brought home weekly reading comprehension tests for which he had to write short answers to questions. Reading comprehension tests were hard for both my kids because, just like in real life, such tests often require drawing connections between someone's feelings and someone's actions. Such social inferences can be hard for young (and old!) ND kids. The "what" questions are easy. The answers to the "why" questions can be hard.

So when Eight would answer all of the questions correctly, he would feel proud of himself. During the semester, he got better and better at it. But even when he provided correct answers, week after week, the teacher would dock his grade 25 percent due to lack of "neatness." The tests came home with 100 percent at the top struck through with ugly red lines, a score of 75 percent written next to it. When Eight handed me his tests, he would cry.

After the umpteenth round of beat-down tears, I asked the teacher for the grading rubric for the quiz. After all, the quiz was supposed to test reading comprehension, not handwriting. And if she's not testing handwriting, then she shouldn't be grading it. And she definitely shouldn't be testing it for any child who has an accommodation that explicitly states not to.

But there was nothing I could do to convince the teacher that my son, despite his intellectual gifts, was never going to have good handwriting. She was too rigid in her beliefs. Because she ignored his accommodations (not just about handwriting), we pulled our son from her class. This is the perpetual struggle of the 2E child, high school student, college student, and adult, and as their parents, it is our job to guide them and stand up for them when they are young. When they are older, it is our job to teach them to stand up for themselves.

TRUSTING YOUR KID

As parents of school-aged ND kids, one of the biggest struggles we face has to do with trusting our kids. We have to trust our kids when they tell us what they need, which can be hard when we have our own expectations about what we want our kids to achieve. We must set aside our own expectations of the path we believe our children should take, which can be very hard.

To learn more about setting aside personal expectations and learning to trust, I interviewed John, a white, cisgender father of a fourteen-year-old neurodivergent daughter.[23] His daughter is twice exceptional and is now homeschooled. John earned his doctorate in biomedical sciences in California and spent many years in an intense career in pharmaceutical start-ups. He met his wife while traveling for work. After living in California for many years, they decided to settle on the East Coast and have their daughter. John continued to do his start-up work after becoming a parent. But, he told me, after his daughter's need became apparent, it felt like "the world punched me in the face and said, 'What you've been doing hasn't been working, and something needs to change.'"

John's preconceptions about his daughter's educational path were influenced by his own childhood education. He grew up in a multigenerational household in the rust belt and was raised by his grandmother, mother, and aunt. His mother had him when she was young, and his father was out of the picture. He told me that because they were very poor, it was very important to his family—and therefore to him—that he do well in school and improve his life. He was a traditionally successful student. He did well in elementary school; for high school, he attended an intense college preparatory Catholic school with a 100 percent college placement rate, going on to his extensive higher education work.

John brought these traditional beliefs about schooling to his parenting style. He told me, "It was apparent when my daughter was young that she was very bright. And I, because of my schooling and my focus, wanted to make sure that she had every opportunity. She had to do basically what I did, right? And my wife was the same way." John's heart, like the hearts of most parents, was in the right place. He said, "If she excelled in school, I thought she would have opportunities outside of our lives, and I wanted her to have that. Personal and professional growth."

Things seemed to pan out the way John and his wife expected when their daughter started school. She did well in elementary school—until she started third grade. She was in an intense magnet program, and by third grade, "she no longer could just keep up by winging it. And she struggled, and she hated it." He now knows that she struggled because of her neurodivergence, which made the arbitrary demands typical of school very difficult for her to manage. "She was being traumatized all along," he said.

John's words are not hyperbole. As psychologist and neurodiversity expert Marcia Eckerd notes, autistic and other neurodivergent kids are frequently traumatized in school. They suffer the "everyday trauma of repeated misunderstanding, invalidation, overstimulation, stress, rejection, and humiliation."[24] As a result, "autistic children come out of school behaving like trauma survivors—distrusting, rejection sensitive, with little or no self-esteem, and diminished as people. They are burdened with a heavy sense of shame and failure that they will hold onto into adulthood."[25]

After being moved to a different elementary school, John's daughter seemed to thrive again. She did so well in fourth and fifth grade that she was invited to a highly selective public middle school for intellectually gifted students. John told me that in her sixth-grade year, the schooling conflict between himself and his daughter came to a head: "My approach to that [gifted] program was different than my daughter's. I viewed it as an opportunity. She viewed it as a pain in the ass. And she rebelled, and that's what led to our crisis. But I didn't see it until the crisis happened, which isn't uncommon." Before realizing his daughter needed support, John told me, "I struggled . . . because my goal was to get her to be rigorous and do the work and show what I knew she was capable of."

John thought school should be "rigorous" in the traditional sense of the word—that is, keeping one's nose to the grindstone, repetitive assignments, high test scores, AP exams, and so on. His daughter had a very different experience, as John told me: "She typically got 100 percent or 0 percent on assignments. If she completed them, she did very well, but she didn't complete most of them." This issue can be traced back to the school's inability to support twice-exceptional children. This lack of support harmed his daughter every day: "She had teachers who were not very empathetic and understanding, and they increased her trauma. I understand now that the teachers had limited bandwidth. . . . They weren't focused on twice-exceptional kids. They were focused on exceptional academic kids, and there was very little support for neurodivergence." John points out, rightly, that teachers are often not to blame for being too overwhelmed to help a 2E kid. Overfull classes, long hours, and poor training are the underlying, institutional causes. We should protect our children and hold people accountable, yes, but understanding the bigger picture helps us be better advocates for our children.

John could tell that his daughter was being traumatized at school. The trauma made her unable to learn, as it would for any ND kid. As John explained, "All of those sensitivities [of his daughter] and all of those mistreatments and trauma, minor traumas and big traumas, are putting kids in a situation where they're never going to learn. People that are anxious and people that feel traumatized do not learn." John told me, "Every ounce of energy goes towards their own survival, or they give up, and they don't survive. . . . It was a very hard thing for me to come around on, appreciating that people genuinely have these sensitivities [like his daughter does, due to neurodivergence], and they genuinely affect their ability to learn and to function."

Once John finally understood that his daughter could not learn in the high-pressure, low-support environment of the gifted public school, he and his wife pulled her from the program to homeschool. By the time they pulled her from school, he was confident that it was the right decision because he had learned to trust that he, and his daughter, knew what was best for her. He explained his thought process to me: "I had to come to the point where I could trust my own instinct, that I know my kid better than any of these so-called professionals. . . . Any given teacher or any given administrator, any given coach . . . all these adults only have a limited time to have a relationship with your child. Maybe one or two years on average. You have a lifetime. So who are you going to trust? . . . Who do you think [knows what] is best for your kid?" But, he said, to reach this conclusion that parents know their kids best, parents must fight against the pressure that teachers, doctors, and other outside authority figures know best.

John transformed from a parent who implicitly trusted teachers and other outsiders to tell him what was right for his daughter's education into someone who knows what is best for her. Now, they have a relationship built on trust; she reaches out to him when she needs help, and he knows that she will do so. He trusts her to make good decisions about her education (which is important for homeschooling, as I discuss later in this chapter). He listens when she speaks, and in turn, she listens to him. I realize these might sound like simple things, but they are crucial to a relationship with a ND kid, especially one who has spent years in a school setting where the adults around them did not take their needs into account.

DISABLING ENVIRONMENTS IN SCHOOLS

What my older son encountered in his third-grade classroom, where the teacher required pristine handwriting, was a "disabling environment." He earned perfect scores on his tests, but the teacher created an arbitrary standard that ensured his failure due to his handwriting disability.

Disability is created by barriers in society: for example, poorly designed transportation and infrastructure, negative stereotyping, and segregation.[26] It is also created, for the purposes of this chapter, by underprepared teachers, understaffed and overcrowded schools, and educators' prejudices about what and how ND and other disabled kids are able to learn. For example, one study revealed that 20 percent of college faculty believe that ND students aren't able to succeed in college.[27] This type of prejudice creates a barrier to success that has nothing to do with neurodiversity. Given this high rate of negative attitudes toward ND college students, it's easy to see why ND students would believe they're better off not outing themselves as ND to professors and instead relinquishing their accommodations. Which is worse? Going without accommodations or risking the prejudice of the professor harming their grade, even if unconsciously?

These social barriers that disabled people face create disabling environments. School is one such disabling environment. If there weren't so many barriers to learning, ND kids would need far fewer accommodations through IEP/504 meetings. Right now we view ND and other disabled students as walking deficits rather than as different types of learners who bring strengths as well as struggles, just like every other student. But knocking down these barriers requires a massive reframing of our thinking about school.

Mainstream schools are frequently a poor choice for neurodivergent children. Autistic psychology researcher Patrick Dwyer explains, with regard to autistic kids, "Many autistic people suffer in mainstream schools. They can be bullied and victimized, isolated and ostracized. They can experience the distress which comes from being in an environment that is hostile to their senses. Their mental health can suffer." Tracking with John's observations of his own daughter's experience, Dwyer points out how this mistreatment itself affects a kid's education: "Some autistic people, in the schools, do not learn the subjects being taught in their curriculum, but helplessness and fear."[28]

Neurodivergent author and activist Jonathan Mooney, in his book *Normal Sucks*, writes about how school created a disabling environment for his dyslexia, rather than one where he could learn and thrive.[29] Because spelling was so hard for him, he states, "I learned to dumb it down. I would write only with words I could copy from around the room. If the word in my head was too long for me to spell, I used a simpler one. When in doubt, I'd scribble a word so no one could read it." There were negative consequences to his coping mechanisms: "I became caught in a full-blown dumb-it-down cycle. My spelling and writing made me feel stupid, so then I was treated as if I was stupid. Then I began to believe I was stupid, and then I began to act stupid, and then—do it all over again the next day."[30] This awful cycle that Mooney describes was created by a school environment where students were allowed to fall through the cracks. In a supportive environment, teachers would have questioned why Mooney was struggling with his writing instead of treating him like he was "stupid" and reinforcing his self-doubt and creating feelings of low self-efficacy and traumatizing him in the process.

Mooney's story is all too familiar to parents of ND kids. Too many kids with learning differences are judged as stupid or delinquent rather than as struggling and in need of help. My own kids attended four schools in six years before we gave up on what we call "outside school" and elected to homeschool instead.

One of the schools they attended was a ghastly expensive "learning center" that touted its ability to teach kids with "learning differences" like mine. My kids attended when they were seven and nine. The school's stated mission "is to transform students with learning differences into confident, independent learners." Each classroom had only three or four students and teachers (supposedly) trained in learning methods to help them. And yet, even in this special school for neurodivergent students, my kids suffered. My younger spent many days banished to the hallway or in the counselor's office because he "refused" to do his work. My older son, who turns inward when he struggles, "refused" in his way, breaking down in tears during class. Parents, beware the word "refuse" from another adult's lips. If your child is refusing to do something, they are suffering. As neurodivergent parent, author, and advocate Heidi Mavir puts it, school refusal is "not a thing."[31] Instead, it is a way for schools to shift blame to parents and kids who are struggling. She writes, "Kids who are healthy and happy and whose needs are being met LOVE school. Kids who are engaged and who feel safe skip into school with a thirst for learning adults marvel at."[32]

One evening, I received an email from Nine's fourth-grade writing teacher. She told me that he "refused" to write during journal time. The writing prompt was this: "If you could have only one wish, what would it be and why?" Earlier that day, when Nine had walked in the door from school, I looked at his face and saw the sadness there. So, I grabbed the dog's leash, and he and I headed right back out the door to take a walk. On dog walks, Nine likes to collect acorns, look for cicada shells, and tell me secrets.

Nine told me all about the writing prompt and how he couldn't do it. "There were just too many wishes," he said. "How could I pick just one?"

Like I do so many times a day, I felt in awe of my child. How, indeed? His sensitive brain had recognized the impossibility of the task. How do you narrow down an infinity of wishes? You can't—it's basic math. If you try to divide infinity by any number, to break infinity down into a manageable amount, you will fail. It will always remain infinity.

"I get it," I said. "I really do."

"I could think of a thousand wishes," he told me, kicking a rock down the sidewalk. "So I couldn't write anything."

He described a painful struggle: how he wanted to wish for all the children to have food, and for all the lost pets to have homes, and for all of the unhappiness in the world to be made happy. My son wishes big, and that's a good thing. There were too many wishes in his head for his teacher's satisfaction but not too many wishes for Nine. And I would never want anyone to suppress that.

Were he a little older, I would have taught him to deliberately wish for more wishes or to wish for Aladdin's lamp. To write, "My wish has five parts, and here is part one." The point is, I would have taught him to consciously rebel in small ways. But I will never teach him to unconsciously obey by squeezing his thoughts into a box too small for them. That boxing in? That's masking. That's how it starts and how it sticks.

I asked Nine what happened after he came up with too many wishes and was unable to write. "She gave me two warnings. And then I started to cry."

I kept my expression clear, but my brain churned. The teacher gave him warnings? Why? At this expensive private school for kids like Nine, in a classroom with only four students and Nine's diagnosis in her brain, couldn't she see that he was suffering, not disobedient?

After the dog walk, I arranged a phone call with Nine's teacher. When we spoke, she was receptive. She meant well. She asked me for strategies for how to work with Nine. In the past week, she told me, the wishes weren't the only roadblock he had run into in writing class. And unlike so many teachers we've had over the years, she listened to me. She didn't act like she knew more about my kid than I did.

Later that day, when I talked to my husband about the phone call, he asked, "What did she say about the warnings, though?"

"She didn't mention those at all."

My husband remained silent, waiting.

"I had to make a choice," I told him.

He agreed, and we both believed we had to make a compromise.

When I tucked Nine into bed that night, he told me that, to make his teacher happy, he decided to wish for a new kitten. I felt a stab of sadness that his school couldn't allow him to be his infinite self, if only in his writing journal. Were they teaching him to write or to conform? Why just one wish, when he had so many to share?

What I learned about Nine and his wishes was this: It doesn't matter how much a school insists they know how to teach your kid. You know your kid best. A teacher might mean well, but meaning well isn't good enough if they see tears as grounds for punishment instead of comfort and curiosity. All week he had struggled with his journal writing, and his teacher couldn't figure out why, when it took me one five-minute dog walk to do so.

A minor adjustment would have allowed her to meet her teaching goal of getting my kid writing in his journal: "Write about what you would wish for. Anything you would wish for." But she couldn't imagine a way to broaden her narrow teaching expectations to allow my kid to thrive, and she traumatized him instead—for an entire week, making him feel worthless, inadequate, deserving of punishment, and humiliated in front of the other children. I could see it in his face: *What is wrong with me, Mom?*

As Anastasia, the mother of a trans ND kid (they/them) who has struggled in multiple schools, told me in an interview, "Why can't they [schools] give us some grace? Show some empathy?"[33] She continued, "In school they demand these things of my kid—show empathy, give grace, show understanding of others. Then we let adults do whatever they want." Frustrated and angry, she told me, "As a result, I don't apologize anymore. If my kid says 'fuck you' to a teacher because she pushes them too far, I don't apologize anymore. . . . I don't have to apologize for my kid anymore, ever."

After so many negative experiences, I have reached the same place as Anastasia. I only wish I reached it sooner. It took another year and a half of painful school and a worldwide pandemic before we started homeschooling our children full time. Hours in the principal's office, the counselor's office, and one suspension. When COVID-19 shut down the schools, the EC teacher at our school told me privately that the services my kids were receiving in public school—we'd left the expensive *learning center* behind—would no longer adequately support our kids. There was just no way the schools could pull it off.

So I activated a homeschool and didn't bother with the online public schooling. When the other kids went back to outside school in person, mine didn't. They had no desire to. Every year we give them a choice, and every year they reject it. They've tasted the freedom of learning things in a way that works for them.

HOMESCHOOLING AND UNSCHOOLING

The requirements for starting a homeschool and maintaining one varies widely state by state. In North Carolina, it is easy to open a homeschool. The creation of the school can all be done online.[34] You file a notice of intent to homeschool and submit a school name and the high school diploma of the teacher (such as a parent). The rest is done on an honor system: Each year, you must fill out a form online stating the name of a standardized test that you have given your children—but you do not need to submit the test results themselves. You must keep records of attendance but do not need to submit those. The state recommends that a homeschool complete instruction for 180 days, but it is only a recommendation. You do not need to submit any lesson plans or completed work. In other states, the requirements are much stricter.

When we first started homeschooling, we started with a rigid curriculum. I was beset by fears that my kids would not learn. That they would "get behind." But more importantly and insidiously, I was afraid that my kids would not learn in a way that was legible to the outside world. Based on my research, I was not alone in these fears. Parents new to homeschooling wonder how their kids will get into college if they don't have materials to show how the kids performed in high school. For months, even years, many homeschool parents cannot let go of fears about their kids' learning progress and their futures. This fear drives parents to make their homeschools mimic outside school, which makes ND children just as miserable as they were in outside school in the first place. The homeschooling parents I spoke with gradually begin to let go and loosen their curriculum, letting their children learn at their own pace and in ways driven by their interests. If you are interested in homeschooling your ND kid, recognize your education choices and think about what is driving them, which is typically fear. Then I recommend finding a local support group for ND homeschoolers and those interested in looser forms of homeschooling and "unschooling."

When I interviewed John, he described his own experience with homeschooling fears to me: "I think it's very common for parents to be fearful that their kids are not conforming to the requirements in school, that they're not developing in an organized way like they should, or that they might miss an opportunity now and never be able to catch up."[35] He also pointed out that the state might instill fear in some parents: "And then even some parents, I think, might be fearful that there are legal requirements for school that they may not be meeting."

Psychologist Peter Gray, in his book on how children learn and the benefits of unschooling, points out what I also found in my anecdotal research: "Most homeschooling parents become increasingly relaxed, less directive, over time." Why? "Both they and their kids typically find the planned curriculum to be boring, so they begin to do more interesting things, usually initiated by the kids." But, Gray points out, in order to let your kids lead their educational experience, you have to trust your children: "With experience, homeschooling parents become increasingly trusting of their children's abilities to direct their own education, and some of them become *unschoolers*."[36]

"Unschooling" was a word I encountered here and there during my homeschool experience, but I didn't start embracing it until recently as my kids grew older—and we started butting heads more. Gray explains unschooling like this: "Defined simply, unschooling is *not schooling*. Unschooling parents do not send their children to school, and at home they do not do the kinds of things that are done at school. They do not establish a curriculum, do not require particular assignments for the purpose of education, and do not test their children to measure progress." So what do these homeschool parents do? Gray writes, "They allow their kids freedom to pursue their own interests and to learn, in their own ways, what they need to know to follow those interests. They believe that learning is a normal part of all life, not something separate that occurs at special times and places."

In her book *Raising Free People: Unschooling as Liberation and Healing Work*, Akilah S. Richards, a Black mother of two daughters who emigrated to the United States from Jamaica when she was a child, defines unschooling a bit differently: "A child-trusting, anti-oppression, liberatory, love-centered approach to parenting and caregiving."[37] Richards's intersectional approach to unschooling reflects the oppression experienced by Black children in schools, where they are forced not only to comply with school norms but also with the racial (white) norms embedded in those school norms. Richards explains how outside schools insist on "studenthood" rather than "personhood," which cannot coexist, as studenthood requires strict obedience and denial of personal needs and self-expression. Richards explains how unschooling is driven by "the core belief that children own themselves and that parents and other adults work with children to nurture their confident autonomy not their ability to obey adults' directives." Outside schools also destroy trust between students and parents, as parents become "extensions of the school system" instead of "allies willing to respect and trust what they were saying." As Richards explains, unschooling teaches "tools for having a healthy relationship to boundaries, to conflict, to communication, to life."[38] As parents of ND kids, we can learn a lot from Richards's approach to unschooling as one of liberation from norms.

But, as Gray points out, unschooling cannot be "the answer for every family, or even most, unless societal changes occur to help support it." Why? Because unschooling, like all homeschooling, "requires a considerable commitment of time and resources." He acknowledges the financial burden, and the sexism, inherent in homeschooling: "Generally, at least one adult has to be home when the kids are young. Most often that adult is the mom, which means that she must be willing to forgo or postpone a career, or able to manage a career from home."[39] But Gray states that these problems are institutional: If our society made a commitment to allow our children to school in a way that fit them best, then every family could afford to homeschool or unschool.

Unfortunately, "school choice" has become a politicized issue, one that is split firmly down party lines. It has become an either/or: To request support for homeschooling means to be against public schools and the public good. But this either/or proposition is a fallacy. The pie of public resources for schools has been deliberately shrunk so small by those who do not care about schools at all that we are all left fighting over the scraps. If there were plenty, then there would be no zero-sum game.

Let's not blame one another in our effort to get all children the education they need. Let's look toward those who defund all efforts to educate as they sit up high watching those of us down in the gladiator pit. There should be money for my children to gain the education they need, for the kids who need public schools for the education they need, and for the rest of the kids out there who need their education, too.

THE TRUST BANK

Long before I had my autism diagnosis but had already been diagnosed with bipolar disorder, I used to joke that I was like a high-end sports car—both high performance and high maintenance. More recently, I gave a talk in which I likened ND people to Formula 1 cars. (Formula 1 racing is one of my intense special interests.) If you watch racing, then you know that F1 cars are the most precise, finely tuned automobiles on the planet. Of the twenty or so cars that start a race, one or two will frequently retire for obscure mechanical reasons—a cooling line here, an electrical connection there. When the announcers talk about track conditions, they speak in terms of one or two degrees of temperature or of tiny bits of detritus on the track. One bit of gravel in the wrong place can wreak havoc on a car. The cars are sensitive to their environment. They are also magnificent. Like with neurodivergence, there is a balance.

Schools struggle with striking a balance when teaching ND kids. Often, a kid's gifts will hide their struggles, or their struggles will hide their gifts. Schools don't know how to make space for a kid who has high support needs but also has some intellectual challenges—or a lot of them. There are two separate tracks, and those tracks do not converge.

But not every parent will have the ability to make the career shift John made to work from home instead of traveling in order to take care of his daughter. Not every parent will be able to homeschool; in fact, most won't. But you can make a shift in mindset to one of trust with your child and belief in your child. If your child comes home from school and tells you about something bad that happened, then you can and must affirm them, listen to them, and comfort them. If a teacher tells you bad things your child has done, always ask your child for their side of the story before making decisions. Don't become an extension of the school, as Richards describes, or you will destroy your trust with your child.

As John told me, "You're either connecting with your child or you're not." The issue, as he has learned, is very black and white. He described to me the metaphor of a "trust bank." He said, "You're either making deposits or making withdrawals." The trick, he told me, is "to always be making deposits."

When a ND kid is crammed into one space or another, they will likely struggle. They may act out in ways that seem disobedient or defiant. Teachers will call parents, and parents will feel guilty and at a loss. Parents may punish their kids to support the school. But you do not have to take teachers as the authority in your kid's life. As John said in his interview, you know your kid best. If your kid is acting out, ask them why. Find out from the teacher what happened before the incident. From there, you can take steps forward that protect your child and address any big issues that might arise.

CHAPTER 6

Bullying, Vulnerability,
and Trauma

In elementary school, there is usually space for kids to be weird and not be singled out for it. When I was eight and nine and ten, I was completely socially oblivious, more so than most kids. But at that age, most kids are still somewhat socially oblivious, so I was still mostly safe from bullying and other unkindnesses.

In fourth grade, during recess, my best friend and I would run along the edge of our school's play field, where the forest met the grass, pretending we were horses. We did not fit in with the other kids, but that was okay. I had an inkling that what we did was weird—there was one girl I remember, a ringleader, who told me one day that I was strange. In fifth grade, I had a different friend, another odd girl, and we did other odd things. But in those early school years, I was mostly oblivious that my social status was perpetually fixed at the fringes of normal.

Unlike other kids, though, unlike even some of my "oddball friends," my social obliviousness did not go away when I entered middle school. Worse, when I turned eleven, I shot up in height, reaching five nine during sixth grade. So while I appeared fourteen, and my intellectual capacity was at high school level or beyond, my social understanding was that of a ten-year-old.

When I walked through the brown double doors of my middle school, I got hit by unspoken rules and regulations that manifested, it seemed, from nothing. These new rules governed every aspect of girls' behavior: clothing, grooming, vocabulary, and, worst of all, for me and others like me, friendship. For the first time, I felt the knife of social wrongness.

Everyone else seemed to know how to dress properly. All the girls wore the same kind of jeans (rolled at the ankles) and the same kind of socks (white, slouchy). I knew I dressed improperly because I was teased, over and over. Sometimes I tried to dress the way the other kids dressed because I thought that my life would be easier if I could fit in just a little. But even when I tried to fit in, I failed.

The girls, I noticed, all wore the same kind of shoes: white, canvas Keds. I wanted a pair, so my mother took me to the store to buy them. The store had Keds in white canvas, but they also had them in white leather, which was shiny and even whiter than the canvas. Picking up the leather Keds, my mom said, "These will stay cleaner." She knew I liked to run outside, playing in our forested backyard. The white canvas shoes, on my adventurous feet, would be covered in stains before the end of the week.

I considered her words. *What difference would it make*, I thought, *wearing white shoes made of leather instead of white shoes made of fabric?* Both had the small blue label at the heel. They were identical in all ways but one.

But when I arrived at school the next day with my new white leather Keds, the girls' words buzzed around me like bees, stinging from all directions.

"Are those even Keds?"

"Do they glow in the dark?"

"They're so bright they hurt my eyes."

The worst were not the girls who were obviously being mean. Obviousness I could decode.

BULLYING, VULNERABILITY, AND TRAUMA   175

No, the worst were the girls who said how much they loved my shoes, how much they wanted a pair.

"Wow, those are the best Keds," one girl said, surrounded by her lunch-table court as I stood holding my tray. "Where did you say you got them?"

I only discovered she was lying because my savvier friend told me later. "She's not being nice to you," she said. "She's making fun of you."

I replayed the encounter in my head, trying to parse the girl's words to find the signs of mockery, the facial expressions that would have given away her true intentions. I couldn't find them.

I went home that day in tears, telling my mother, "These shoes are wrong." All the pent-up pain from being teased, the tears I refused to shed at school, came out at home, the place that was supposed to be safe. "They made fun of me," I said, sobbing.

"Don't be ridiculous," my mom said. "They're just Keds."

I tried to explain, but she wouldn't listen. She began the refrain that I would hear all through middle school, all through high school, all through my twenties and thirties: "Everyone gets teased, Katie. You're not special." It's true that many kids get teased and bullied, but not to the same degree as ND kids.[1] For someone like me, it was harder to fit in, harder to even get my leather Keds in the door.

Between the girls at school and my mom at home, I learned a valuable lesson. Even if I tried to follow all the rules, fitting in was going to be much harder for me to do. The rules were too obscure and complicated and too hard for me to decode. Friendship was a minefield, and I would always come through injured. And if I did get injured, my injuries would not garner sympathy at home.

Better to not follow the rules at all. Better to act like I did not care. So I hid my differences behind indifference. That was the mask I put on, and few people were allowed to see behind it— for decades.

But I knew early on that I didn't want that pain for my kids. I wanted them to recognize bullies and to have the self-assurance to stand up to them. I wasn't sure how to teach them these things that were never taught to me. But I decided I wouldn't gaslight them, telling them that they weren't the target of bullies or of other mistreatment when they told me that they were. I would never tell them that they were ridiculous for being sad.

No, I promised myself that would protect them when they couldn't protect themselves, that I would believe and affirm them, and that I would find resources to teach them how to protect themselves, even if the teacher couldn't be me.

The bullying of my own kids started early, in pre-K. I couldn't believe how early it started. My older kid would come home in tears, telling me about the other kid at school, Rex, who targeted him on the playground. I took his reports seriously, immediately meeting his teachers. The teachers agreed with my son's recounting of what was happening and told me they were taking action.

One day, as I was picking up my kid from pre-K, I saw Rex with his mother in the parking lot. She was bent at the waist, finger pointing in his small, pale face, and I saw terror in his eyes. Then, as fast as a striking snake, she slapped him across his face. Standing by my car, I flinched at the cracking sound.

For a moment, I despaired. The truth about bullies is that they are not born, they're made. How can I despise a child who is torturing my own when his own suffering is so heartbreaking? I could not.

It turned out that dropping my hate of bullies was an important lesson. Because I didn't hate bullies, I didn't teach my children to hate them, either. I taught them to love themselves instead and pity those whose only pleasure is in making people suffer. I also learned to recognize that the problem wasn't the bullies, it was the systems that enabled them.

When my older son was six years old, I got a call from school, where he was in first grade. The principal told me that Six had broken the rules at lunch by sharing food with another kid. The rule was in place, I knew, to protect children who might have allergies, and I respected it.

Because Six was food sensitive, I sent him to school with packed lunches of food he loved, along with extra money to buy a carton of milk and one of the "treats," food we never had at home. Six always bought Doritos, his favorite. He was in trouble, the school told me, because he was giving his Doritos to another kid.

I thought, *Why would he give his favorite snack away?* It made no sense.

Later, I asked Six that question. He started crying. He told me that another boy in his class, Ace, was making him give away his treats.

"How?" I asked Six.

"He said he would poison me."

Ice washed over my body. "Tell me more," I said, in the calmest voice I could muster.

"He has a vial of poison, and he'll poison me if I don't give him my Doritos."

"Why didn't you tell me?" I asked.

My son cried harder. "He'll poison me if I tell anyone."

Hugging him, I promised him that he was safe because I would protect him and that I was safe too because I was too strong for Ace. Then I made an appointment with the principal.

The next day at the meeting, I told the principal about Ace threatening Six with poison.

"But the poison isn't real, right?" the principal said.

"That's right," I said, wondering why she was asking me such an obvious question.

"So it's just your son's imagination."

At her words, I knew that something was about to go very wrong. I said, "The words Ace is saying are not my son's imagination."

The principal pushed back. "But he plays with Ace at recess."

My hands started to shake. I could picture Ace holding court at recess, the charismatic class bully and all of his acolytes, with my son in the dangerous borderlands, trying to navigate the safest path through the unstructured time.

"If you say so," I replied.

"Here's what I think," she said. "I think your son is fantasizing."

I drew a sharp breath. *Fantasizing what?* I said, "So you aren't going to do anything about Ace?"

She waved her hand. "We've already separated them at lunch because your son broke the food-sharing rule."

Heart racing, I left. My kid was being bullied, and the school wasn't going to do anything about it. Worse, he was the one being punished.

So, I controlled what I could—my kid's sense of safety. From then on, we talked explicitly about bullies: how it is always safe to share things with his parents, how *no one* is stronger than his mom, and how it is my number one job to keep him safe. To this day, if you ask my teenaged kids, "What is your mom's number one job?," they will reply in unison, "To keep me safe." What they don't remember is how that call-and-response started. It didn't start because of kidnappers or fires or speeding cars. It started because of bullies. They have haunted us all since we stepped out into the world. They are integral to the life of a neurodivergent kid—and to the life of schools.

WHO IS VULNERABLE?

In the United States, 15–28 percent of children are bullied each school year.[2] Psychologists define bullying as "a type of aggression that is (a) intended to harm others, (b) repetitive, and (c) characterized by an imbalance of power between the perpetrator and victim."[3] The purpose of bullying is to gain dominance and social status. Because an imbalance of power is inherent in bullying, bullies target certain kids because they know that they have more power over those victims. Bullies also tend to have strong social skills.[4] In recent years, kids who are chronically bullied are more likely to attempt or commit suicide.[5]

All disabled kids (including neurodivergent kids) are up to four times more likely to be bullied than abled kids.[6] Research that has studied students in "special education" and their interaction with their general education peers "found that children with disabilities who are easily provoked or visibly bothered by verbal taunts and teasing are frequently targeted for acts of physical and verbal aggression."[7] Stories of bullied ND kids abound. My kids have experienced bullying in outside school; indeed, bullying is one of the reasons we chose to homeschool. In his book *Normal Sucks*, ND advocate and author Jonathan Mooney, who has dyslexia and ADHD, talks about how, when he was in elementary school and learning to read, he was ashamed of the early reader books he had to use because "the other kids would taunt: 'Jonathan, go back to the dumb reading group.'"[8]

Other research has found that a lack of "social competency" increased the risk of bully victimization in kids. In this context, "social competence refers to the ability to regulate one's emotions and to maintain positive interpersonal relationships with others."[9] These studies were not focused on ND kids but rather the population of children as a whole. However, ND kids tend to struggle with social skills, emotional regulation, and interpersonal relationships.[10]

Of all disabled kids, ND kids are the most likely to be bullied because of their difficulty interacting with their peers. In one study of bullying and disability, those with ADHD and "emotional disturbance" were most frequently chronically bullied. Note that emotional disturbance is not a diagnosis but rather a category under the Individuals with Disabilities Education Act. It encompasses a variety of traits, such as "an inability to build or maintain satisfactory interpersonal relationships with peers and teachers," "inappropriate types of behavior or feelings under normal circumstances," and "general pervasive mood of unhappiness or depression."[11] Another study showed that the highest levels of bully victimization were kids with ADHD, autism, and learning disabilities.[12] Finally, one study compared the victimization rates for neurotypical and autistic adolescents.[13] The national bully rate for autistic kids was 46.3 percent compared to the rate for the general adolescent population, which was 10.6 percent. In short, "emotional and behavioral difficulties are the most significant indicators of chronic victimization risk, followed by history of prior victimization and low socioeconomic status."[14] Worse, the bullying of disabled kids tends to be chronic. One study showed that, once a disabled student had been bullied, their risk of repeated bully victimization increased 500 percent over the six-year study period.[15]

However, the language with which researchers describe bullying of ND kids is problematic. One recent study noted that kids with "symptoms" that create "difficulty reading and responding appropriately to social situations" will "invite" themselves to be bullied because they fail to follow social norms or regulate their emotions properly.[16] This language, in particular the term "invite," blames the victim for causing themselves to be bullied. One bullying research study divided bullying victims in multiple types. One type is the "provocative" victim, who "exhibits poor social behaviors that irritate or annoy others, thereby eliciting bullying."[17] In school, these victims typically have poor concentration, lack impulse control, and disrupt classrooms. According to this study, because the "provocative victim" is annoying, they draw the bully's attention to themselves.

Just like the language of invitation, the word "provoking" blames victims of bullying—even if the researchers did not intend to do so but only to classify or describe. However, in the minds of readers, the words "invite" and "provoke" imply fault on the part of the victim. Even expert readers are not immune to the weight these words carry. In no interpretation of the English language do the words "provoke" and "invite" mean anything other than to cause the harm that comes your way. Research studies that replicate the same victim-blaming language over decades also circulate into presentations at teacher conferences. The language then circulates among workers in the teaching profession. Finally, it makes its way into a parent-school conference, one with a parent desperate to protect her son from a bully, who is then told by the school that her son provoked it—an experience I have had more than once.

Scientists are growing more aware that the way studies are framed and the language they use affect their outcomes.

(In turn, the outcomes of studies affect the policies that they manifest.) Kids with ADHD are already seen as "problem" kids in schools: Teachers see them as disruptive and distracted and don't want them in their classrooms. If these studies show that they're so annoying that they "invite" bullies to target them, then adults will not see it as their duty to protect them. Similarly, autistic kids are overly sensitive to foods, or sounds, or clothing. They have routines that cause them great distress when they are disrupted. Their lack of social savvy causes them to talk about strange interests without realizing that others don't want to listen. These behaviors "provoke" bullying, right? Of course not.

When my kid reported to me that another kid would poison him if he didn't hand over his Doritos, my kid believed that he and I were in real danger. The bully physically threatened him, even if the bully didn't use his fists. He was able to threaten my kid because mine was less socially savvy. As the principal said to me, and as I agreed, of course the other kid didn't actually have poison. But that was not the point. In fact, under North Carolina law (and the law of the land in the United States), verbal threats of bodily harm to you or someone you love that are intended to instill fear, especially with the intent to control or manipulate, are criminal assault.[18] The law protects against not just actual violence (poisoning) but against the fear and dread that a person feels because of the threat of violence ("I will poison you if you do not do what I say").

The socially savvy bully identified my kid's weakness—his naivete—and exploited it to steal his food for weeks, terrifying him so much that he was too afraid to tell me because my life would be in danger, too. In fact, the bully kept my son in such terror that he was too afraid to ask for help from anyone. And then, in the end, my victimized son was the one who was punished. In the eyes of the principal, he was to blame for his own victimization. The lineage of this punishment and blame can be traced back to research that says ND kids are irritating and annoying and "invite" and "provoke" mistreatment.[19] As I wrote earlier in this book, how we *talk* about neurodivergent people affects how we *treat* neurodivergent people.

BULLYING PATTERNS IN SCHOOL

To learn more about how bullying affects young people into adulthood, I interviewed Amanda, a professor of disability studies at a public university in the southeastern United States.[20] Amanda is a white, cisgender woman who is bisexual. She was diagnosed with OCD (obsessive-compulsive disorder), anxiety, and depression during childhood. She was diagnosed as ADHD in graduate school and also with PTSD because of the ongoing trauma she experienced in childhood. She told me that, during her elementary and middle school years, because of her neurodivergence, "I was horribly, horribly, bullied." She attended a nice private school at the time, but the school offered her little protection. During a game of tug-of-war in school, she was pushed to the ground and got rope burns. She broke her coccyx because "I was running away from bullies when I was on roller skates and had an accident." She sustained multiple concussions that led to chronic migraines. After the migraines started, she would have to go to the nurse at school to get her migraine medicine, and the medicine would put her to sleep. While she was asleep in the nurse's office, she was sexually assaulted. She didn't share the assaults with her parents, though, because she had trouble remembering them for a long time.

When she shared the bullying with her parents, her parents didn't want to cause any sort of uproar. This lack of parental advocacy is not unusual, as parents are frequently afraid to make waves, either in the school or in their community. But Amanda's parents were particularly afraid to make waves. She told me, "We tried to talk to the school. . . . The thing is, [my parents] wanted to keep me in this private school because it was a good school." Eventually, though, the bullying got so bad that her parents moved her to a public school when she was twelve. Everything was fine for a while, but then the bullying started again. To avoid the bullies, she would hide in the bathroom, "because I was so scared of something happening to me." Soon, she told me, "I started developing an eating disorder because the bullies told me I was fat. And then I started also developing some self-harm behaviors. Mainly stuff that wouldn't leave huge marks. I would pinch myself. My mom would find scratches, and I'd just say I scratched myself at night." She also started pulling out her own hair. She told me, "Everything came to a head when I was fourteen. . . . There was a kid who had started bullying me again . . . and that set off the alarm bells that this is starting again. And a couple of days later was my first major suicide attempt."

Amanda wasn't formally diagnosed with OCD, anxiety, and depression until her sophomore year of high school, but she suffered at the hands of bullies from an early age because of her neurodivergences. She finally escaped bullies her junior and senior years of high school when she was able to take most of her classes online and handpick the ones she took in person, selecting only the kindest teachers and avoiding the ones who treated her poorly because of her neurodivergences. She also received regular therapy and medical care.

But the years of trauma she suffered as a child led to a diagnosis of PTSD as an adult, which is not unusual for former ND kids because of the amount they suffer as young people.[21]

Indeed, it doesn't take much research to learn that Amanda's story is not an unusual one. As parents, we must build trust with our children to encourage them to share with us when they are being bullied. Then we must believe them when they tell us what is happening and do everything we can to protect them—and not stop until they are safe.

ADULTS VICTIMIZING CHILDREN

Victimization of ND kids is perpetrated not only by other kids but also by adults. Every day, parents put their children into the care of adults (and quasi-adults), expecting that their children will be cared for and safe. But bullying by adults is not uncommon, especially if the children are neurodivergent. Earlier in this book, I described the bullying of my younger child by adult coaches during the two days he spent on our neighborhood swim team. In one instance, a coach yanked my six-year-old from the pool after a minor, unintentional infraction and yelled in his face, "What is wrong with you?," in front of the other kids. My son replied, "I forget things," and started crying.

The coach's "question" was of the rhetorical variety—in her eyes, there was indeed something wrong with my son. But being a highly literal ND six-year-old, my son answered her question anyway. In doing so, he felt deeply ashamed. Because of incidents like this, he believed, for a long time afterward, that something was indeed wrong with him. What we didn't realize was just how many incidents like this one he'd had to endure: at school, at camps, even with extended family members. We are still encountering the lingering trauma from wounds inflicted by adults that he has encountered in his short life, and most neurodivergent kids suffer similar wounds from adults in their lives. These wounds leave lasting trauma that manifests as unhealthy behaviors in adulthood. As ADHDer and neuro-diversity advocate Dani Donovan wrote on Instagram, "Children who are constantly criticized grow into teens who learn to hate themselves for failing to live up to others' expectations who grow into adults who reflexively over-apologize because they have been conditioned to believe they are always disappointing everyone."[22]

According to psychologists, the mistreatment of children can be studied at a societal level. In *Free to Learn*, psychologist Peter Gray describes societal-level violence this way: "Research involving many types of societies has shown systematic relationships between a society's structure and its treatment of children. The more violent a society was overall, the more likely it was that parents used corporal punishment. The beating of children correlated positively with the frequencies of wife beating, harsh punishment of criminals, wars, and other indices of societal violence." In the United States, we glorify the harsh punishment of criminals and war, and we turn our backs on domestic violence. Gray explains other factors that lead to the abuse of children: "It also correlated strongly with the degree of social stratification in society. The greater the differentiation in power among people in a society, the more frequent the use of corporal punishment by parents." What do kids learn from this punishment? Gray explains, "Parents use corporal punishment ultimately to teach their children to respect the hierarchy of power. Some people are more powerful than others and must be obeyed, no questions asked."[23]

In a society like ours, with strong social stratification based on wealth and other factors, adults are more likely to use violence to punish children. It is also important to recognize that violence can be verbal, not just physical. This authoritarian violence, whether physical or verbal, insists that children comply with social norms—in our society's case, the hierarchy of power. This hierarchy places the normal above the abnormal, the neurotypical above the neurodivergent.

When they are outside of their homes, kids spend a large amount of time in the care of teachers. Neurodivergent children can be unsafe in the care of teachers because ableism causes teachers to fail to take care of ND kids. In one research study, 45 percent of teachers report having bullied a student.[24] Also, teachers tend to avoid protecting victims who fail to display "normal" emotional responses to being bullied. For example, when some students disclosed being bullied to teachers, the "teachers sometimes described [the] children's experience of being bullied as the child misperceiving the situation"—which might happen more often with ND kids who are less socially savvy.[25] Teachers withhold support from a victim if they believe the victim did not "deserve" the teacher's support because the student was to blame for being victimized. Other studies show that ND students are frequently blamed for being victimized because they are "irritating."[26] Teachers make assumptions about victimized students that influence their responses to them, such as whether a student is "well adjusted" or "passive or lacking in confidence."[27] If a child does not look like a victim, then the teacher will not believe the child is a victim at all. For example, if a victim responds to bullying with anger, then the teacher may tend to blame the victim for being victimized. If the victim appears confident, then the teacher may tend to avoid intervening.

There are many problems with these adult presumptions about what a victim should look like. Among them is the fact that ND kids frequently present reactions outside the norm when they are in tough situations. They may shut down and seem unexpectedly calm. Because of emotional dysregulation, they may explode in anger or melt down. They may act aloof as a protective device. The point is that because ND kids may not present as "normal" when bullied, they therefore may not gain the same support from adults who witness them being bullied or when the kids themselves report it. They may be told that they are imagining things, that they are bringing it on themselves, or any of the other things that adults say to minimize the experience of victimized kids. This minimization is in itself another type of victimization. Children learn that they cannot go to adults for help, and they feel isolated and alone. This is a tragic outcome because research shows how beneficial it is for children to be able to ask adults for help. In a study about adult responses to bullying, researchers note, "When children are listened to [about victimization], they can make peace with their negative experience and create a positive narrative, which can be associated with having a good later life."[28]

Sometimes it isn't easy to spot when an adult is harming a neurodivergent kid. The teacher doesn't realize it because they think they're doing the right thing. We, as parents, must educate ourselves about our kids and then stand up for them. To learn more about how teachers can influence parents, I interviewed John, a white, cisgender married father of a fourteen-year-old neurodivergent daughter. His daughter is twice exceptional and now homeschooled.[29] When his daughter was in third grade, her parents did not realize that she was neurodivergent. They only knew that she was struggling in school both academically and socially, despite her excellent grades in first and second grade. John related being called in for a conference with the principal, the vice principal, and his daughter's teachers. When they told him that his daughter was struggling, the teacher said, "I know what to do. I just need to push her over the wall." In other words, the teacher believed that all John's daughter needed was more pressure.

At the time, John didn't know about his daughter's neurodiversity and how to collaborate with her. Despite his ignorance about his daughter's specific needs, he remembered hearing the teacher's words and thinking, "This is a kid who has, who currently does, and who has always loved school. She used to get up in the morning, and she couldn't wait to go to school." But she didn't feel that way anymore. John realized that if the teacher continued to push his daughter while she was struggling emotionally, "she's not only going to hate you, she's going to hate me." In our interview, John emphasized over and over that, as parents, we know our children better than their coaches, teachers, and even doctors and therapists do. We have to stand up for them against other adults and listen to our inner voices that tell us when things aren't right.

In another story about this same school and teacher, John told me that when his daughter started to really struggle academically, she would bring books to school to read at lunch and recess. The teacher told John that his daughter "removes herself from peer interactions" with the books. The teacher said, "I feel like she needs those peer interactions. So at lunch I now forbid her from reading books." The teacher did the same during recess. John told me how much this edict harmed his daughter because she "just took the one thing that is [the daughter's] outlet." His daughter "was clearly traumatized, and I know that now. Because the books were what was keeping her safe, and the teacher removed that safety net." John's wisdom about his daughter's needs didn't come all at once, just like mine didn't and yours likely won't either. We are all constantly learning what our children need to feel safe and how to protect them from adults who are supposed to protect them but fail to do so. We must trust our instincts and our children. And we must be vigilant, as things can change from time to time and stage to stage. As our ND children grow and change, so do their surroundings. Developing a set of tools we can fall back on to navigate those changes is important and will vary according to your child's needs, your resources, and the cooperation of those around you.

WHAT CAN WE DO AS PARENTS?

It can be hard to hear this, but as parents, we victimize our neurodivergent kids. We don't even realize we're doing it. My own parents didn't realize they were bullying me when they told me to stop crying on Christmas morning because I became overwhelmed and dysregulated. We do it when we tell our children that they have to eat certain foods, wear certain clothes, or stop doing their favorite things because they need to "branch out." We do it when we tell them that they talk too much or talk too much about only one thing. We hurt them when we say that they're not allowed to play with only one friend; no, they must make other friends, too. They must tie their shoes (instead of wearing slip-on sneakers), they must wear button-down shirts (instead of pull-on shirts), and wear pants that button and zip (instead of pull-on pants) because, darn it, that's what they'll have to do in the real world, right? So why can't they do it now? With all of these words and actions, we are telling our kids that because they are different or have needs that we refuse to meet, something is wrong with them. Worse, we are teaching our kids that they can't trust us to keep them safe.

We all do it, in large ways and small, because we are immersed in ableist social norms. Even parents with abled children fall back on the easy method of telling their kids to *just do what they are told*. Parents of ND kids, though, face a constant battle to push back against those norms, especially the ones that have infected our own brains. The pressure to conform attacks in sneaky ways, such as this: We want our kids to be happy, right? Of course we do. And, ever since we ourselves were small, the world has told us, whether we are neurodivergent or not, that the only way to be happy is to eat, dress, talk, and behave "normally." Without even realizing it, we bring social surveillance into our homes, with us as its enforcers and our children as its victims.

One sly way parents try to normalize their ND kids' behavior is when we tell our kids that the victimization that they experience outside the home isn't as bad as they say it is. We tell them that they're overreacting or that "all kids hate middle school." Autistic author and advocate Jennifer Cook O'Toole recounts this type of victimization by her mother in her memoir, *Autism in Heels*. When she was in middle school, O'Toole danced with a traveling ballet troupe. She was three years younger than the rest of the girls and autistic as well—ripe for victimization. In a hotel room while the troupe was traveling, as she took her turn in the hotel shower, the older girls opened the door, turned off the lights, and dumped a bucket of ice over the shower curtain, laughing the entire time. O'Toole recounts how unsafe she felt: "Stunned, I stood shaking in the dark and began to cry. I just wanted my mom." But her mom didn't provide comfort; she provided the opposite, telling her, "Maybe it was a joke . . . just playing around." This lack of affirmation is common among parents of bullied children. It tells the child that they are alone, with no adult to keep them safe. O'Toole continues, "But I knew it wasn't [a joke]. I'd danced since I was two. Had been invited to come to the school for the performing arts. It was my passion.

My soul. Now, I couldn't stop shaking. I'd made them hate me, too. I'd just been me. I'd been naked. And that day, dance became another place to scare me. To hurt me."[30] In this story, O'Toole was victimized by the older girls in her dance group who targeted her for her autistic behavior. Then, she was victimized again by her mother, who failed to affirm her experience.

When our kids tell us that they've been victimized, believe them. Let them tell us their stories. We must understand that bullying is *not* the same for ND kids as it is for all other kids. This might be hard to square with your personal experience, but our ND kids do indeed have it worse. As I wrote earlier in this chapter, psychological research shows that "emotional and behavioral difficulties are the most significant indicators of chronic victimization risk," in particular the behaviors related to ADHD and autism.[31] Furthermore, bullying of ND kids tends to be chronic and last for years.[32] School administrators and other leaders fail to protect ND kids from bullying, blaming them for "provoking" it with their irritating behavior.[33] They also fail to protect ND kids from bullies because they don't respond to bullying the way most neurotypical kids do.[34]

What can we do to protect our ND kids at school? We must advocate for them in school, even if it feels fruitless, so that our kids know that we will fight for them and so that the schools know that we are watching out for our kids. In addition to meeting with teachers and administrators, we can file reports at the school district level and ensure that an investigation takes place. You can use your child's IEP to request goals to protect your kid, such as "improve self-advocacy skills," "learn how to report unsafe behavior," and "gain ability to identify a bully."

In her memoir, O'Toole tells stories about how her mother casually victimized her by pointing out that her ND behavior provoked negative interactions. O'Toole writes that she suffered "a lifetime of comments . . . in which people I loved harshly criticized my social skills." Her mother "made up stories with my Cabbage Patch Kids in which the redhead was a bossy smartypants whom no one really liked; the blonde doll as cute, likable, and funny—everyone's favorite. Did I mention my mom was blonde?"[35] Another time, her mom asked her, "Why doesn't anyone you want to be friends with want to be friends with you?"[36] O'Toole's mother was influenced by ableist social norms that taught her to believe that her daughter's behavior was defective and that the best way to fix her daughter was through constant criticism. This criticism caused lifelong scars. Books like O'Toole's can help parents of ND kids understand how to do better by our children.

We can also help our children by changing our own behavior. For example, we can gain a better understanding of where seemingly "negative" behaviors are coming from and avoiding victimizing our kids when they act in these ways. As autistic author and parenting expert Amanda Diekman points out, "Contrary to popular belief and common parenting practice, children are hardwired to please their adults, and do not lack motivation to do the right thing."[37] If your ND child is not tying their shoes, it isn't because they are rebelling, even if it they are acting like they are—for example, by expressing anger. Instead of punishing your child for their supposed failure, *ask* them why they aren't doing the thing you've requested. Once the pressure is off and your child feels safe, you might hear some quiet words they were too ashamed to tell you when you were angry: "I don't know how to tie them."

It can be difficult for a kid who is anxious and stressed out to admit to a weakness or ask for help, especially if they are so far gone into the bad-emotion spiral that they are dysregulated and melting down or if they are afraid of being punished for the weakness. As Diekman writes, "The basic assumption underlying punishment and reward parenting is that kids need to be incentivized to do the right thing." But, Diekman points out that this assumption is false: "Brain science shows that children actually need parents who stay attuned and connected through all their challenging behaviors and powerful emotions." That is, when your child is struggling, punishment is the last thing they need. Indeed, "having a connected adult is the most essential factor in children's long-term health and positive development."[38]

In my interview with John, he shared a lot of information about how to parent a ND kid without pressuring them to conform to imaginary standards.[39] John is a master of connected parenting. He told me, "You're supposed to tell your kids what you want and have them conform. That's the 'should-supposed-to' world of the parenting manual." But, John points out, this parenting style is not only flawed, it is dangerous. Teaching children to conform in every situation puts them at risk of trying to please everyone and comply with outside instructions instead of listening to themselves. John told me, "If you teach your child, especially a girl, to conform to what you want, what do you think they're going to be like when they grow up? Do you want them to conform to every male they meet? . . . Are you kidding me, right? You can't raise them like that." He gave me some advice he'd heard along the way: "If you act like a tyrant in your household, then you can expect a revolt one day. Because it always happens." As John points out, teaching kids to rigidly conform is also a matter of safety for our kids. Neurodivergent kids are already vulnerable to bullying and other forms of victimization. Teaching them to conform to everything any adult tells them to do, to rigidly obey hierarchy, sets them up to be victimized even more.

Instead, as parents of ND kids, we must teach our children that they need to follow those rules that protect them and others, adhere to the values of our family and the community, and always be themselves and find those people who accept them as they are. This parental work is both a duty and a gift. Our duty is to learn all we can about how to be better parents. Our gift is that we get to watch our kids grow under parenting that allows them to flourish.

Acknowledgments

Thank you to my team at Johns Hopkins University Press, especially my editor, Suzanne Staszak-Silva, who ushered this book into the world. And thank you to my friend and fellow author Rebecca Pope-Ruark, who encouraged me to find a home for my book at Hopkins Press in the first place.

Thank you to my early readers, Bronwyn Charlton, Lauren Faulkenberry, Sarah McInnes, and Ayla Samli. They read many chapters of this book, some of them multiple times, and gave excellent feedback.

Thank you to my writing partners, Alexa Chew, Lauren Faulkenberry, Rachel Del Grosso, and Darci Swisher, for helping me stay on pace to make my deadlines.

Thank you to Wildacres Retreat for welcoming me with a writer's residency where much of this book was written.

Thank you to my author squad, Camille Pagán and Kelly Harms, who provide a steady stream of humor and support as we navigate our careers.

Thank you to Nicole Chung, my editor first at *The Toast* and then at *Catapult*, for helping me start writing for the public in the first place over a decade ago, for showing me that writing about one's neurodivergent child can be done with grace and respect, and for editing my "Mom, Interrupted" column, which was the inspiration for this book.

Thank you to all the individuals who agreed to be interviewed for this book and who shared their wisdom with me.

Thank you to my family. My parents let me pester them with questions about my childhood. They also fielded very serious phone calls from me whenever I was in crisis about my own children after something terrible happened to them. My parents may not care when my dishwasher breaks and floods my kitchen, but when my kid gets kicked off the swim team, they're ready to set something on fire. The best thing you can receive from your kids' grandparents is the confidence that they would do *anything* to keep your children safe and happy.

Thank you to my sister Chris and her family, who are always kind and loving; we're so glad to have you live down the street. Thank you to my sister Janet for being the big sister I need and to Mimi Carol, my aunt and, more importantly, my kids' great-aunt, teacher, and supporter.

Thank you to my colleagues in the field of disability studies. Although we might not see each other at conferences anymore, and even if we haven't met in person, knowing you are out there doing good work is an inspiration for me to keep going:

Alice Wong (and the Disability Visibility Project)

Catherine Denial

Catherine Prendergast

Claire McGuire

Ellie Margolis

Eric Garcia

Jordynn Jack

Katherine Macfarlane

Keith Myers

Kevin Gannon

Lee Skallerup Bessette

Margaret Price

Porochista Khakpour

Rebecca Pope-Ruark

Remi Yergeau

Rick Godden

Shannon des Roches Rosa (and the *Thinking Person's Guide to Autism*)

Stephanie Kerschbaum

Temple Grandin (who endorsed this book when it was still an unrevised Word document)

The Cyborg Jill Weise

And so many more.

Thank you to the adults who have touched the lives of me and my children and helped shape who we are today.

The people who have helped guide my kids as they've grown:

Alec Moore

Max Fritsch

Mike Mills

Josh Collins

Hatcher Williams

Jessica Maloney

Christine Denny

Ms. Goerne

Ms. Dixon

Mr. Courtney

Ms. Nelson

Macy Williamson

Jim Bedford

Piper Jones

Jenna Smith

Melissa Daeschner

Kalin Fraker Mason

Santiago Arenas

Bev Burnette

Melissa Davis

Mindy and her dad, Larry

Clare Baxter

Kylo Balan

Robert Buxton

Jil Christensen

And the people who guided me:

Connie Kotis

Quint Barefoot

Mrs. Roberts

Mrs. Parrish

Diana L. Dell

Marla Wald

Terri Galant

Andy Crichton

Mary Oliver

Tom Sleigh

And finally, thanks to the two teenagers who found me on the beach when I was three years old after I wandered off for an hour and my parents were convinced that I had drowned. Like most ND children, I've always taken my own path, and we all need the kindness of others to help us on our way.

Notes

Preface

1. Nicole Chung, "The Worry I No Longer Remember Living Without," *Hazlitt*, March 9, 2017, https://hazlitt.net/feature/worry-i-no-longer -remember-living-without.

2. Katie Rose Guest Pryal, "The World Doesn't Bend for Disabled Kids (or Disabled Parents)," *Catapult*, July 10, 2018, https://perma.cc/ZX2L -JX9E.

3. Aaden Friday, "When You're Autistic, Abuse Is Considered Love," *The Establishment*, March 21, 2018, https://theestablishment.co/when -youre-autistic-abuse-is-considered-love-84eea4011844/index.html.

4. Pryal, "The World Doesn't Bend for Disabled Kids."

Introduction

1. Katie Rose Guest Pryal, *The Freelance Academic: Reclaim Your Career, Creativity, and Mental Health*, 2nd ed. (Chapel Hill, NC: Blue Crow Books, 2024).

2. Katie Rose Guest Pryal, "Life of the Mind Interrupted," a column, *The Chronicle of Higher Education*, from 2014 to 2017.

3. Rebecca R. Winters, Jamilia J. Blake, and Siqi Chen, "Bully Victimization Among Children with Attention-Deficit/Hyperactivity Disorder: A Longitudinal Examination of Behavioral Phenotypes," *Journal of Emotional and Behavioral Disorders* 28, no. 2 (2020): 80–91, https://doi.org/10.1177 /1063426618814724.

4. Meng-Chuan Lai and Simon Baron-Cohen, "Identifying the Lost Generation of Adults with Autism Spectrum Conditions," *The Lancet Psychiatry* 2, no. 11 (2015): 1013–27, https://doi.org/10.1016/S2215 -0366(15)00277-1.

5. Inhwan Park, Jared Gong, Gregory L. Lyons, Tomoya Hirota, Michio Takahashi, Bora Kim et al., "Prevalence of and Factors Associated with School Bullying in Students with Autism Spectrum Disorder: A Cross-Cultural Meta-Analysis," *Yonsei Medical Journal* 61, no. 11 (2020): 909–22, https://doi.org/10.3349/ymj.2020.61.11.909.

6. Julie Lounds Taylor and Katherine O. Gotham, "Cumulative Life Events, Traumatic Experiences, and Psychiatric Symptomatology in Transition-Aged Youth with Autism Spectrum Disorder," *Journal of Neurodevelopmental Disorders* 8 (2016): article 28, https://doi.org/10.1186/s11689-016-9160-y.

7. Board of Education of the Hendrick Hudson Central School District v. Rowley, 458 U.S. 176 (1982).

8. Mark Galliver, Emma Gowling, William Farr, Aaron Gain, and Ian Male, "Cost of Assessing a Child for Possible Autism Spectrum Disorder? An Observational Study of Current Practice in Child Development Centres in the UK," *BMJ Paediatrics Open* 1, no. 1 (2017): e000052, https://doi.org/10.1136/bmjpo-2017-000052.

9. Katharine E. Zuckerman, Brianna Sinche, Angie Mejia, Martiza Cobian, Thomas Becker, and Christina Nicolaidis, "Latino Parents' Perspectives of Barriers to Autism Diagnosis," *Academic Pediatrics* 14, no. 3 (2014): 301–8, https://doi.org/10.1016/j.acap.2013.12.004.

10. Laura Foran Lewis, "Exploring the Experience of Self-Diagnosis of Autism Spectrum Disorder in Adults," *Archives of Psychiatric Nursing* 30, no. 5 (2016): 575–80, https://doi.org/10.1016/j.apnu.2016.03.009.

11. Brené Brown, *Daring Greatly: How the Courage to Be Vulnerable Transforms the Way We Live, Love, Parent, and Lead* (New York: Avery, 2015), 24.

12. Brown, *Daring Greatly*, 24.

13. Lennard J. Davis, "Introduction: Normality, Power, and Culture," in *The Disability Studies Reader*, 4th ed. (New York: Taylor & Francis, 2013), 1.

14. Davis, "Introduction," 3.

15. Davis, "Introduction," 3.

16. Davis, "Introduction," 5.

17. Davis, "Introduction," 1.

18. Davis, "Introduction," 5.

19. Jonathan Mooney, *Normal Sucks: How to Live, Learn, and Thrive Outside the Lines* (New York: Henry Holt, 2019).

20. Mooney, *Normal Sucks*, 18.

21. R. George and M. A. Stokes, "Sexual Orientation in Autism Spectrum Disorder," *Autism Research* 11, no. 1 (2018): 133–41, https://doi.org/10.1002/aur.1892.

22. Kala Allen Omeiza, *Autistic and Black: Our Experiences of Growth, Progress, and Empowerment* (London: Jessica Kingsley Publishers, 2024), 11.

23. Talia Hibbert, *Get a Life, Chloe Brown* (New York: Avon, 2019); Bassey Ikpi, *I'm Telling the Truth, but I'm Lying: Essays* (New York: Harper Perennial, 2019); Rivers Solomon, *An Unkindness of Ghosts* (New York: Akashic Books, 2017).

24. Lydia X. Z. Brown, Letters to the Revolution: Letters of Inspiration to Those Targeted by the Upcoming Administration, 2017, http:// www.letterstotherevolution.com/lydia-x-z-brown; Helen Hoang, *The Heart Principle* (Thorndike, ME: Center Point, 2021); Esmé Weijun Wang, *The Collected Schizophrenias: Essays* (Minneapolis, MN: Graywolf Press, 2019).

25. Eric Garcia, *We're Not Broken: Changing the Autism Conversation* (Boston: Houghton Mifflin Harcourt, 2021).

26. Meghan Ashburn, Jules Edwards, and Morénike Giwa Onaiwu, *I Will Die on This Hill: Autistic Adults, Autism Parents, and the Children Who Deserve a Better World* (London: Jessica Kingsley Publishers, 2023). Jules Edwards is a neurodivergent Anishinaabe writer.

27. Rita George and Mark A. Stokes, "Gender Identity and Sexual Orientation in Autism Spectrum Disorder," *Autism* 22, no. 8 (2018): 970–82, https://doi.org/10.1177/1362361317714587; Reubs J. Walsh, Lydia Krabbendam, Jeroen Dewinter, and Sander Begeer, "Brief Report: Gender Identity Differences in Autistic Adults: Associations with Perceptual and Socio-Cognitive Profiles," *Journal of Autism and Developmental Disorders* 48, no. 12 (2018): 4070–78, https://doi.org/10.1007/s10803-018-3702-y.

28. Judy Singer, "'Why Can't You Be Normal for Once in Your Life?': From a 'Problem with No Name' to the Emergence of a New Category of Difference," in *Disability Discourse*, ed. Mairian Corker and Sally French (Philadelphia, PA: Open University Press, 1999).

29. Rosemarie Garland-Thomson, *Extraordinary Bodies: Figuring Physical Disability in American Culture and Literature* (New York: Columbia University Press, 2017), 8.

30. Katie Rose Guest Pryal, *A Light in the Tower: A New Reckoning with Mental Health in Higher Education* (Lawrence: University Press of Kansas, 2024).

31. Eric B. Elbogen and Sally C. Johnson, "The Intricate Link Between Violence and Mental Disorder: Results from the National Epidemiologic Survey on Alcohol and Related Conditions," *Archives of General Psychiatry* 66, no. 2 (2009): 155, https://doi.org/10.1001/archgenpsychiatry.2008.537. Elbogen and Johnson write, regarding their message research project, "Multivariate analyses confirmed that severe mental illness alone did not

significantly predict committing violent acts; rather, historical, disposi-
tional, and contextual factors were associated with future violence."

32. Katie Rose Guest Pryal, "Accommodations and Accessibility:
What's the Difference?," *Psychology Today*, November 6, 2023, https://
www.psychologytoday.com/intl/blog/living-neurodivergence/202310
/accommodations-and-accessibility-whats-the-difference.

33. Pryal, "Accommodations and Accessibility."

34. Andrew Solomon, *Far from the Tree: Parents, Children and the Search
for Identity* (New York: Scribner, 2012).

35. Hannah Belcher, "Autistic People and Masking," National Autistic
Society (UK), July 7, 2022, https://perma.cc/68PT-E2N2.

36. Devon Price, *Unmasking Autism: Discovering the New Faces of
Neurodiversity* (New York: Harmony, 2022).

Chapter 1. The Exclusion of Neurodivergent Kids from Public Life

1. Substance Abuse and Mental Health Services Administration, *DSM-5
Changes: Implications for Child Serious Emotional Disturbance* (Rockville,
MD: National Center for Biotechnology Information, 2016), 16, https://
www.ncbi.nlm.nih.gov/books/NBK519712/.

2. Substance Abuse and Mental Health Services Administration, *DSM-5
Changes*, 16.

3. Grace W. Gengoux, "Priming for Social Activities: Effects on Interactions Between Children with Autism and Typically Developing Peers,"
Journal of Positive Behavior Interventions 17, no. 3 (2015): 182, https://doi.org
/10.1177/1098300714561862.

4. Pete Wharmby, "A Personal Perspective: How Special Interests Can
Help Autistic Students Thrive," National Autistic Society (UK), October 14,
2022, https://www.autism.org.uk/advice-and-guidance/professional
-practice/special-interests.

5. Pete Wharmby, *What I Want to Talk About: How Autistic Special
Interests Shape a Life* (London: Jessica Kingsley Publishers, 2022).

6. Susan E. Longtin, "Using the College Infrastructure to Support
Students on the Autism Spectrum," *Journal of Postsecondary Education
and Disability* 27, no. 1 (2014): 63–72.

7. Kathleen D. Viezel, Elizabeth Williams, and Wesley H. Dotson,
"College-Based Support Programs for Students with Autism," *Focus on
Autism and Other Developmental Disabilities* 35, no. 4 (2020): 234–45,
https://doi.org/10.1177/1088357620954369.

8. Suneeta Kercood, Janice A. Grskovic, Devender Banda, and Jasmine Begeske, "Working Memory and Autism: A Review of Literature," *Research in Autism Spectrum Disorders* 8, no. 10 (2014): 1317, https://doi.org/10.1016/j .rasd.2014.06.011.

9. "Why Are Memories Attached to Emotions So Strong?," Columbia University Irving Medical Center, July 13, 2020, https://www.cuimc .columbia.edu/news/why-are-memories-attached-emotions-so-strong.

10. Sophia, interview with "Sophia" (a pseudonym, real name on file with author), video chat, July 9, 2024.

11. "Varying Support Needs," National Autistic Society (UK), accessed December 17, 2023, https://www.autism.org.uk/advice-and-guidance /what-is-autism/varying-support-needs.

12. Claire Jack, "From Autistic Linear Spectrum to Pie Chart Spectrum," *Psychology Today*, August 16, 2022, https://www.psychologytoday.com/us /blog/women-autism-spectrum-disorder/202208/autistic-linear-spectrum -pie-chart-spectrum.

13. Cameron, interview with "Cameron" (a pseudonym, real name on file with author), video chat, July 17, 2024.

14. Anastasia, interview with "Anastasia" (a pseudonym, real name on file with author), video chat, July 5, 2024.

Chapter 2. Previewing, Meltdowns, and Social Policing

1. Megan Anna Neff, "The Autistic and ADHD Nervous System," Neurodivergent Insights, accessed August 21, 2024, https://perma.cc/2LLE -MZFA.

2. Gengoux, "Priming for Social Activities," 182.

3. Sarah L. Chellappa, "Neuroaffirming Services for Autistic People," *The Lancet Psychiatry* 11, no. 2 (2023): 96–97, https://doi.org/10.1016/S2215 -0366(23)00405-4.

4. Aaron R. Dallman, Kathryn L. Williams, and Lauren Villa, "Neurodiversity-Affirming Practices Are a Moral Imperative for Occupational Therapy," *The Open Journal of Occupational Therapy* 10, no. 2 (2022): 1–9, https://doi.org/10.15453/2168-6408.1937.

5. Michelle Grenier and Pat Yeaton, "Previewing: A Successful Strategy for Students with Autism," *Journal of Physical Education, Recreation and Dance* 82, no. 1 (2011): 28, https://doi.org/10.1080/07303084.2011 .10598558.

6. Gengoux, "Priming for Social Activities," 184.

7. Jessie Mewshaw, interview with Jessie Mewshaw, pediatric speech and language pathologist, email, June 14, 2024.

8. "Social Stories," Head Start, US Department of Health and Human Services, March 31, 2023, https://eclkc.ohs.acf.hhs.gov/children-disabilities/article/social-stories.

9. Dori Zener, "Journey to Diagnosis for Women with Autism," *Advances in Autism* 5, no. 1 (2019): 5, https://doi.org/10.1108/AIA-10-2018-0041.

10. Amanda Diekman, *Low-Demand Parenting: Dropping Demands, Restoring Calm, and Finding Connection with Your Uniquely Wired Child* (Philadelphia: Jessica Kingsley Publishers, 2023), 24.

11. Diekman, *Low-Demand Parenting*, 25.

12. Laura Foran Lewis and Kailey Stevens, "The Lived Experience of Meltdowns for Autistic Adults," *Autism* 27, no. 6 (2023): 1817–25, https://doi.org/10.1177/13623613221145783.

13. Hannah Gadsby, *Ten Steps to "Nanette": A Memoir Situation* (New York: Ballantine, 2022), 272.

14. Gadsby, *Ten Steps*, 272.

15. Gadsby, *Ten Steps*, 272.

16. Price, *Unmasking Autism*, 34.

17. Jennifer Cook O'Toole, *Autism in Heels: The Untold Story of a Female Life on the Spectrum* (New York: Skyhorse Publishing, 2018), 136.

18. Sara Ryan, "'Meltdowns', Surveillance and Managing Emotions: Going Out with Children with Autism," *Health and Place* 16, no. 5 (2010): 868, https://doi.org/10.1016/j.healthplace.2010.04.012.

19. Ryan, "Meltdowns," 868.

20. Ryan, "Meltdowns," 868.

21. Ryan, "Meltdowns," 869.

22. Ryan, "Meltdowns," 868–69.

23. Ryan, "Meltdowns," 869.

24. Ryan, "Meltdowns," 873.

25. Ryan, "Meltdowns," 873.

26. Ryan, "Meltdowns," 874.

27. Ryan, "Meltdowns," 874.

28. Ryan, "Meltdowns," 874.

29. Adrienne Hurst, "Black, Autistic, and Killed by Police," *Chicago Reader*, December 17, 2015, http://chicagoreader.com/news-politics/black-autistic-and-killed-by-police/.

30. Kala Allen Omeiza, *Autistic and Black: Our Experiences of Growth, Progress, and Empowerment* (London: Jessica Kingsley Publishers, 2024).

31. Sophia, interview.

32. Price, *Unmasking Autism*, 8.

33. Deirdre Atkinson-Byrne, "Receiving Gifts—An Autistic Experience," *inTune Pathways Blog*, December 7, 2022, https://www.kristyforbes.com.au /blog/receiving-gifts-an-autistic-experience.

34. Kerem Coskun and Yücel Oksuz, "Impact of Emotional Literacy Training on Students' Emotional Intelligence Performance in Primary Schools," *International Journal of Assessment Tools in Education* 6, no. 1 (2019): 36–47, https://doi.org/10.21449/ijate.503393.

35. "Fostering Emotional Literacy in Young Children: Labeling Emotions," Head Start, US Department of Health and Human Services, accessed June 25, 2024, https://eclkc.ohs.acf.hhs.gov/mental-health /article/fostering-emotional-literacy-young-children-labeling-emotions.

36. "Mixed Emotions Game," Play Therapy Supply, accessed June 26, 2024, https://www.playtherapysupply.com/games/mixed-emotions.

37. Ryan, "Meltdowns," 874.

Chapter 3. Masking, Treatments, and Affirming Neurodiversity

1. Renée M. Green, Alyssa M. Travers, Yamini Howe, and Christopher J. McDougle, "Women and Autism Spectrum Disorder: Diagnosis and Implications for Treatment of Adolescents and Adults," *Current Psychiatry Reports* 21, no. 4 (2019): 22, https://doi.org/10.1007/s11920-019-1006-3.

2. Lai and Baron-Cohen, "Identifying the Lost Generation of Adults."

3. Price, *Unmasking Autism*, 36.

4. Price, *Unmasking Autism*, 100.

5. Felicity Sedgewick, Vivian Hill, and Elizabeth Pellicano, "'It's Different for Girls': Gender Differences in the Friendships and Conflict of Autistic and Neurotypical Adolescents," *Autism* 23, no. 5 (2019): 1119–32, https://doi.org/10.1177/1362361318794930.

6. Julia Cook, Laura Crane, Laura Hull, Laura Bourne, and William Mandy, "Self-Reported Camouflaging Behaviours Used by Autistic Adults During Everyday Social Interactions," *Autism* 26, no. 2 (2022): 406–21, https://doi.org/10.1177/13623613211026754.

7. Paul R. Sterzing, Paul T. Shattuck, Sarah C. Narendorf, Mary Wagner, and Benjamin P. Cooper, "Bullying Involvement and Autism Spectrum Disorders: Prevalence and Correlates of Bullying Involvement Among Adolescents with an Autism Spectrum Disorder," *Archives of Pediatrics and Adolescent Medicine* 166, no. 11 (2012): 1058, https://doi.org /10.1001/archpediatrics.2012.790.

8. *The Big Bang Theory*, 2007–19, on CBS.

9. *Hannibal*, 2013–15, on NBC.

10. A. X. Rutten, R. R. J. M. Vermeiren, and Ch. Van Nieuwenhuizen, "Autism in Adult and Juvenile Delinquents: A Literature Review," *Child and Adolescent Psychiatry and Mental Health* 11 (2017): 45, https://doi.org/10.1186/s13034-017-0181-4.

11. Grace Trundle, Katy A. Jones, Danielle Ropar, and Vincent Egan, "Prevalence of Victimisation in Autistic Individuals: A Systematic Review and Meta-Analysis," *Trauma, Violence and Abuse* 24, no. 4 (2023): 2282–96, https://doi.org/10.1177/15248380221093689.

12. *Community*, 2009–15, on NBC / Yahoo Screen.

13. Kate Ellis, "How Watching Abed Nadir Made Me Feel Seen," *The McGill Daily*, April 5, 2021, https://www.mcgilldaily.com/2021/04/watching-abed-nadir-watching-myself/.

14. Cook et al., "Self-Reported Camouflaging Behaviours."

15. Renée M. Green et al., "Women and Autism Spectrum Disorder: Diagnosis and Implications for Treatment of Adolescents and Adults," *Current Psychiatry Reports* 21, no. 4 (March 9, 2019): 22, https://doi.org/10.1007/s11920-019-1006-3.

16. Cook et al., "Self-Reported Camouflaging Behaviours," 407.

17. Price, *Unmasking Autism*, 8.

18. Price, *Unmasking Autism*, 8.

19. Price, *Unmasking Autism*, 9.

20. Steven K. Kapp, Robyn Steward, Laura Crane, Daisy Elliott, Chris Elphick, Elizabeth Pellicano et al., "'People Should Be Allowed to Do What They Like': Autistic Adults' Views and Experiences of Stimming," *Autism* 23, no. 7 (2019): 1782–92, https://doi.org/10.1177/1362361319829628.

21. Lisa Jo Rudy, "What Is Stimming?," Verywell Health, updated October 16, 2022, https://www.verywellhealth.com/what-is-stimming-in-autism-260034.

22. Kapp et al., "People Should Be Allowed," 1783.

23. Boon Yen Lau, Ruth Leong, Mirko Uljarevic, Jian Wei Lerh, Jacqui Rodgers, Matthew J. Hollocks et al., "Anxiety in Young People with Autism Spectrum Disorder: Common and Autism-Related Anxiety Experiences and Their Associations with Individual Characteristics," *Autism* 24, no. 5 (2020): 1111–26, https://doi.org/10.1177/1362361319886246.

24. Jennifer S. Baldwin and Mark R. Dadds, "Examining Alternative Explanations of the Covariation of ADHD and Anxiety Symptoms in

Children: A Community Study," *Journal of Abnormal Child Psychology* 36, no. 1 (2008): 67–79, https://doi.org/10.1007/s10802-007-9160-1.

25. Lisa Jo Rudy, "Autism Terms You May Be Misunderstanding," Verywell Health, August 21, 2023, https://www.verywellhealth.com/common-autism -terms-you-may-be-misunderstanding-4058516.

26. Rudy, "Autism Terms."

27. Sophia, interview.

28. Lisa Jo Rudy, "Examples of Stimming," Verywell Health, August 18, 2024, https://www.verywellhealth.com/what-is-stimming-in-autism -260034.

29. Rudy, "Examples of Stimming."

30. Price, *Unmasking Autism.*

31. Ryan, "Meltdowns."

32. Heidi Mavir, *Your Child Is Not Broken: Parent Your Neurodivergent Child Without Losing Your Mind* (London: Bluebird, 2023), 35.

33. Mavir, *Your Child Is Not Broken*, 26–27.

34. Food and Drug Administration, "FDA Warns Consumers About the Dangerous and Potentially Life Threatening Side Effects of Miracle Mineral Solution," news release, August 12, 2019, https://www.fda.gov /news-events/press-announcements/fda-warns-consumers-about -dangerous-and-potentially-life-threatening-side-effects-miracle -mineral.

35. Britta Lokting, "A Controversial Autism Treatment, Feuding Parents, and the Two Sons Stuck in the Middle," *Jezebel*, August 4, 2020, https://jezebel.com/a-controversial-autism-treatment-feuding-parents -and-1843923786.

36. Michael Davidson, "Vaccination as a Cause of Autism—Myths and Controversies," *Dialogues in Clinical Neuroscience* 19, no. 4 (2017): 403–7.

37. "HBOT Treatment for Autism: A Promising Alternative," National Hyperbaric Treatment Center, accessed July 5, 2024, https://www.national hyperbaric.com/hbot-treatments-and-conditions/autism.

38. Justyna Podgórska-Bednarz and Lidia Perenc, "Hyperbaric Oxygen Therapy for Children and Youth with Autism Spectrum Disorder: A Review," *Brain Sciences* 11, no. 7 (2021): 916, https://doi.org/10.3390/brain sci11070916.

39. "A Mother's Fight Against Court-Ordered ABA," NeuroClastic, July 4, 2019, https://neuroclastic.com/mothers-aba-experience/.

40. Emily Sohn, "Low Standards Corrode Quality of Popular Autism Therapy," *The Transmitter: Neuroscience News and Perspectives*, October 28, 2020, https://www.thetransmitter.org/spectrum/low-standards-corrode -quality-popular-autism-therapy/.

41. "Applied Behavior Analysis (ABA)," Autism Speaks, accessed July 5, 2024, https://www.autismspeaks.org/applied-behavior-analysis.

42. Meghan Ashburn and Jules Edwards, *I Will Die on This Hill: Autistic Adults, Autism Parents, and the Children Who Deserve a Better World* (London: Jessica Kingsley Publishers, 2023).

43. "Applied Behavior Analysis."

44. Price, *Unmasking Autism*, 100.

45. Jessie Mewshaw, interview with Jessie Mewshaw, pediatric speech and language pathologist, video chat, June 28, 2024.

46. American Medical Association House of Delegates, *Revision of H-185.921, Removal of AMA Support for Applied Behavior Analysis*, April 3, 2023, https://www.ama-assn.org/system/files/a23-706.pdf.

47. Price, *Unmasking Autism*, 36.

48. "ABAI Finally Opposes the Use of Electric Shocks at the JRC," Autistic Self-Advocacy Network, November 16, 2022, https://autisticadvocacy.org /2022/11/abai-finally-opposes-the-use-of-electric-shocks-at-the-jrc/.

49. Henny Kupferstein, "Evidence of Increased PTSD Symptoms in Autistics Exposed to Applied Behavior Analysis," *Advances in Autism* 4, no. 1 (2018): 19–29, https://doi.org/10.1108/AIA-08-2017-0016; Aileen Herlinda Sandoval-Norton, Gary Shkedy, and Dalia Shkedy, "How Much Compliance Is Too Much Compliance: Is Long-Term ABA Therapy Abuse?," *Cogent Psychology* 6, no. 1 (2019): 1641258, https://doi.org/10.1080 /23311908.2019.1641258.

50. Brian Reichow, Kara Hume, Erin E. Barton, and Brian A. Boyd, "Early Intensive Behavioral Intervention (EIBI) for Young Children with Autism Spectrum Disorders (ASD)," *Cochrane Database of Systematic Reviews*, no. 5 (2018), https://doi.org/10.1002/14651858.CD009260.pub3.

51. Amy Grant, "ABA Therapy and PTSD," Therapist Neurodiversity Collective, March 3, 2021, https://therapistndc.org/aba-therapy-and-ptsd/.

52. US Department of Defense, *The Department of Defense Comprehensive Autism Care Demonstration Quarterly Report to Congress Second Quarter, Fiscal Year 2019*, October 25, 2019, https://www.altteaching.org/wp-content /uploads/2019/11/TRICARE-Autism-Report.pdf?x55003.

53. Chellappa, "Neuroaffirming Services for Autistic People"; American Medical Association House of Delegates, *Revision of H-185.921*.

54. Justin Barrett Leaf, Robert K. Ross, Joseph H. Cihon, and Mary Jane Weiss, "Evaluating Kupferstein's Claims of the Relationship of Behavioral Intervention to PTSS for Individuals with Autism," *Advances in Autism* 4, no. 3 (2018): 122–29, https://doi.org/10.1108/AIA-02-2018-0007.

55. Kathryn A. Gorycki, Paula R. Ruppel, and Thomas Zane, "Is Long-Term ABA Therapy Abusive: A Response to Sandoval-Norton and Shkedy," *Cogent Psychology* 7, no. 1 (2020): 1823615, https://doi.org/10.1080/23311908.2020.1823615.

56. Catherine Lord and Tameika Meadows, "How to Know If You're Getting Good ABA," Child Mind Institute, accessed July 7, 2024, https://childmind.org/article/know-getting-good-aba/.

57. Cameron, interview.

58. "How We Embrace Neuro-Affirming ABA Practice," Adventures with Autism, accessed July 22, 2024, https://adventureswithautism.net/f/how-we-embrace-neuro-affirming-aba-practice.

59. Mavir, *Your Child Is Not Broken*, 40.

60. C. L. Lynch, "Invisible Abuse: ABA and the Things Only Autistic People Can See," NeuroClastic, March 28, 2019, https://neuroclastic.com/invisible-abuse-aba-and-the-things-only-autistic-people-can-see/.

61. Elizabeth Devita-Raeburn, "The Controversy over Autism's Most Common Therapy," *The Transmitter: Neuroscience News and Perspectives*, August 10, 2016, https://www.thetransmitter.org/spectrum/controversy-autisms-common-therapy/.

62. Jordynn Jack, *Autism and Gender: From Refrigerator Mothers to Computer Geeks* (Urbana: University of Illinois Press, 2014), 30.

63. Gadsby, *Ten Steps to "Nanette,"* 270.

64. C. L. Lynch, "Invisible Abuse."

65. Mewshaw, interview.

66. Ryan, "Meltdowns," 873–74.

67. Omeiza, *Autistic and Black*, 123.

68. Omeiza, *Autistic and Black*, 52.

69. Tiffany "Tiffy" Hammond, "A Journey in Masking," *Fidgets and Fries*, April 20, 2024, https://tiffywrites.substack.com/p/a-journey-in-masking.

70. Mewshaw, interview.

Chapter 4. The Medication Double Bind

1. *The Bling Ring*, directed by Sofia Coppola (A24, 2013).

2. Gadsby, *Ten Steps to "Nanette,"* 266.

3. Daniel F. Connor, "Problems of Overdiagnosis and Overprescribing in ADHD," *Psychiatric Times* 28, no. 8 (2011), https://www.psychiatrictimes .com/view/problems-overdiagnosis-and-overprescribing-adhd.

4. Connor, "Problems of Overdiagnosis."

5. Conner, "Problems of Overdiagnosis."

6. Natasha Brown, Margaret McLafferty, Siobhan M. O'Neill, Rachel McHugh, Caoimhe Ward, Louise McBride et al., "The Mediating Roles of Mental Health and Substance Use on Suicidal Behavior Among Undergraduate Students with ADHD," *Journal of Attention Disorders* 26, no. 11 (2022): 1437–51, https://doi.org/10.1177/10870547221075844.

7. Brown et al., "The Mediating Roles of Mental Health and Substance Use," 1446.

8. Brown et al., "The Mediating Roles of Mental Health and Substance Use," 1446.

9. Barbara G., interview with Barbara G. (full name on file with author), in person, November 2022.

10. "DSM History," American Psychiatric Association, accessed July 14, 2024, https://www.psychiatry.org:443/psychiatrists/practice/dsm/about -dsm/history-of-the-dsm.

11. Anastasia, interview.

12. Sophia, interview.

13. Elbogen and Johnson, "The Intricate Link Between Violence and Mental Disorder," 152.

14. Wendy Wisner, "Suicide and Bipolar Disorder: Symptoms, Treatment, and Prevention," Healthline, July 26, 2022, https://www.healthline .com/health/suicide-and-bipolar.

Chapter 5. School Accommodations

1. Individuals with Disabilities Education Act of 2004, 20 U.S.C. § 1400.

2. Kyrie E. Dragoo and Eric Lomax, *The Individuals with Disabilities Education Act: A Comparison of State Eligibility Criteria* (Congressional Research Service of the United States Government, October 12, 2020), https://crsreports.congress.gov/product/pdf/R/R46566.

3. Individuals with Disabilities Education Act of 2004, 20 U.S.C. § 1400.

4. Board of Education of the Hendrick Hudson Central School District v. Rowley, 458 U.S. 176 (1982).

5. Individuals with Disabilities Education Act of 2004, 20 U.S.C. § 1400.

6. Individuals with Disabilities Education Act of 2004, 20 U.S.C. § 1400.

7. Autism Society of North Carolina, *The IEP Toolkit*, Rev.5.14 (Raleigh: Autism Society of North America), 3, accessed July 23, 2024, https://www .autismsociety-nc.org/wp-content/uploads/IEP-Toolkit-web-links.pdf.

8. Autism Society of North Carolina, *The IEP Toolkit*, 3.

9. Rehabilitation Act of 1973, 29 U.S.C. § 701.

10. Sharon Schultz, "Differences Between a 504 Plan and an Individualized Education Program (IEP)," National Education Association, December 2022, https://www.nea.org/professional-excellence/student -engagement/tools-tips/differences-between-504-plan-and-individualized -education-program-iep.

11. Schultz, "Differences Between."

12. Autism Society of North Carolina, *The IEP Toolkit*.

13. Schultz, "Differences Between."

14. Katie Rose Guest Pryal, "What Is the Invisible Burden of School Accommodations?," *Psychology Today*, June 11, 2024, https://www .psychologytoday.com/intl/blog/living-neurodivergence/202406/what-is -the-invisible-burden-of-school-accommodations.

15. Anthony, interview with "Anthony" (a pseudonym, real name on file with author), video chat, July 15, 2024.

16. Emily King, interview with Emily King, PhD, about IEP/504 plan advocacy, email, August 2, 2024.

17. Cameron, interview.

18. Arwa K. Nasir, Whitney Strong-Bak, and Marie Bernard, "Diagnostic Evaluation of Autism Spectrum Disorder in Pediatric Primary Care," *Journal of Primary Care and Community Health* 15 (2024): 21501319241247997, https://doi.org/10.1177/21501319241247997.

19. "School-to-Prison Pipeline," Autistic Self-Advocacy Network, June 2022, https://autisticadvocacy.org/wp-content/uploads/2022/06 /School-to-Prison-Pipeline-PL.pdf.

20. "School-to-Prison Pipeline."

21. Linda E. Brody and Carol J. Mills, "Gifted Children with Learning Disabilities: A Review of the Issues," *Journal of Learning Disabilities* 30, no. 3 (1997): 282–83, https://doi.org/10.1177/002221949703000304.

22. Anthony, interview.

23. John, videochat interview with "John" (a pseudonym, real name on file with author), July 6, 2024.

24. Marcia Eckerd, "Are Autistic Students Traumatized in School?," Association for Autism and Neurodiversity, November 3, 2022, https://

aane.org/autism-info-faqs/library/are-autistic-students-traumatized-in
-school/.

25. Eckerd, "Are Autistic Students Traumatized?"

26. "Definitions of Disability," Disability Information Bureau (UK), accessed July 23, 2024, https://www.dibservices.org.uk/definitions
-disability.

27. Thomas J. Tobin and Kirsten T. Behling, *Reach Everyone, Teach Everyone: Universal Design for Learning in Higher Education*, 1st ed. (Morgantown: West Virginia University Press, 2018).

28. Patrick Dwyer, "Who to Include? Who to Exclude?," Autistic Scholar, August 11, 2018, http://www.autisticscholar.com/who-to-include.

29. Mooney, *Normal Sucks.*

30. Mooney, *Normal Sucks*, 17.

31. Mavir, *Your Child Is Not Broken*, 26.

32. Mavir, *Your Child Is Not Broken*, 26–27.

33. Anastasia, interview.

34. "Home School Requirements and Recommendations," North Carolina Department of Administration, accessed July 24, 2024, https://
www.doa.nc.gov/divisions/non-public-education/home-schools
/requirements-recommendations.

35. John, interview.

36. Peter Gray, *Free to Learn: Why Unleashing the Instinct to Play Will Make Our Children Happier, More Self-Reliant, and Better Students for Life* (New York: Basic Books, 2013), 227.

37. Akilah S. Richards, *Raising Free People: Unschooling as Liberation and Healing Work* (Oakland, CA: PM Press, 2020), 11–12.

38. Richards, *Raising Free People*, 5.

39. Gray, *Free to Learn*, 230.

Chapter 6. Bullying, Vulnerability, and Trauma

1. Jamilia J. Blake, Eun Sook Kim, Emily M. Lund, Qiong Zhou, Oi-man Kwok, and Michael R. Benz, "Predictors of Bully Victimization in Students with Disabilities: A Longitudinal Examination Using a National Data Set," *Journal of Disability Policy Studies* 26, no. 4 (2016): 199, https://
doi.org/10.1177/1044207314539012.

2. Blake et al., "Predictors of Bully Victimization," 199.

3. Winters et al., "Bully Victimization," 80.

4. Winters et al., "Bully Victimization," 81.

5. Blake et al., "Predictors of Bully Victimization," 199.

6. Blake et al., "Predictors of Bully Victimization," 199.

7. Cathy Evans and Donna Eder, "'No Exit': Processes of Social Isolation in the Middle School," *Journal of Contemporary Ethnography* 22, no. 2 (1993): 139–70, https://doi.org/10.1177/089124193022002001.

8. Mooney, *Normal Sucks*, 16.

9. Paul Caldarella and Kenneth W. Merrell, "Common Dimensions of Social Skills of Children and Adolescents: A Taxonomy of Positive Behaviors," *School Psychology Review* 26, no. 2 (1997): 264–78, https://doi.org/10.1080/02796015.1997.12085865.

10. Blake et al., "Predictors of Bully Victimization," 200.

11. Individuals with Disabilities Education Act of 2004, 20 U.S.C. § 1400, Sec. 300.8 (c) (4), Emotional Disturbance, https://sites.ed.gov/idea/regs/b/a/300.8/c/4/.

12. Winters et al., "Bully Victimization," 81.

13. Sterzing et al., "Bullying Involvement and Autism Spectrum Disorders," 1058.

14. Winters et al., "Bully Victimization," 81.

15. Blake et al., "Predictors of Bully Victimization," 204.

16. Blake et al., "Predictors of Bully Victimization," 200.

17. Winters et al., "Bully Victimization," 81.

18. "What Is Considered a Threat In NC? Legal Protection Against Domestic Violence," Plekan Law, May 13, 2024, https://plekanlaw.com/what-is-considered-a-threat-in-nc-legal-protection-against-domestic-violence/.

19. Winters et al., "Bully Victimization," 81.

20. Amanda, interview with "Amanda" (a pseudonym, real name on file with author), video chat, July 5, 2024.

21. Eckerd, "Are Autistic Students Traumatized?"

22. Dani Donovan, "Children Who Are Constantly Criticized," Twitter/X, December 19, 2019, https://x.com/danidonovan/status/1204029540068134912.

23. Gray, *Free to Learn*, 49.

24. Stuart W. Twemlow and Peter Fonagy, "The Prevalence of Teachers Who Bully Students in Schools with Differing Levels of Behavioral Problems," *American Journal of Psychiatry* 162, no. 12 (2005): 2387–89, https://doi.org/10.1176/appi.ajp.162.12.2387.

25. Ylva Bjereld, Kristian Daneback, and Faye Mishna, "Adults' Responses to Bullying: The Victimized Youth's Perspectives," *Research Papers in Education* 36, no. 3 (2021): 259, https://doi.org/10.1080/02671522.2019.1646793.

26. Winters et al., "Bully Victimization," 80.

27. Winters et al., "Bully Victimization," 80.

28. Bjereld et al., "Adults' Responses to Bullying."

29. John, interview.

30. O'Toole, *Autism in Heels*, 141.

31. Winters et al., "Bully Victimization."

32. Blake et al., "Predictors of Bully Victimization," 204.

33. Winters et al., "Bully Victimization."

34. Winters et al., "Bully Victimization," 81.

35. O'Toole, *Autism in Heels*, 132.

36. O'Toole, *Autism in Heels*, 143.

37. Diekman, *Low-Demand Parenting*, 22.

38. Diekman, *Low-Demand Parenting*, 22.

39. John, interview.

Index

2E (twice exceptional, 129, 130, 153–56, 159, 171
504 plans, 138, 142, 145–52. *See also* IEPs (individualized education programs)

ABA (Applied Behavior Analysis), 88, 101–9
Abed Nadir (*Community* character), 91–92
abled, as term, 19–20
ableism: and accommodations, 49; defined, 20, 31; internalized, 16–17, 20, 31, 87, 89, 90, 92–93; and masking, 16–17, 92–93; as narrow-minded, 41–45; and neurodivergence as "fake," 116; of parents, 31, 87; and social norms, 16–17, 70, 190–95; ubiquity of, 20; and unsolicited advice, 116, 134
accessibility, 20–21
accommodations: and ableism, 49; *vs.* accessibility, 21; and advocacy by parent, 137–42, 146, 147–49, 156, 170–72; and advocates, hired, 147–49; and college, 13, 161; costs, 140, 150; defined, 20–21; described, 142–48; 504 plans, 138, 142, 145–52; IEPs, 138, 142–52; ignoring of, 155–56; and legal counsel, 140, 147–49; and not being disabled "enough," 153–55, 171; as overshadowing gifts, 138–39, 153, 171; process of, 146–49; and race, 150–52; and socioeconomic status, 150; and sons of author, 138–39; and 2E kids, 129, 153–56, 159, 171
ADA (Americans with Disabilities Act), 19
Adderall, 120, 121, 127

ADHD (attention deficit hyperactivity disorder): and author, 124–25; and bullying, 180; defined, 7; and executive function, 38; medication, 4, 116, 120–23, 131–32; and mental health, 94, 123; and neurodivergence as "fake," 120–23; and sons of author, xvi, 2, 7, 99, 126, 127, 138; stigma of, 120–23; teachers' dislike of, 182; treatments and therapies, 99, 106; under/overdiagnosis, 121–23
adults: and authority, 35; blame and belittling by, 37, 41; bullying by, 126, 127, 176–78, 185–95; and Christmas, 57–58, 78–79, 190; conformity as benefiting, 44, 46; and culture of scarcity, 11–15, 49–50, 54; impatience with neurodivergent kids, 2, 6–9, 11; masking as benefiting, 78–79; neurodivergent adults and schism over treatment, 105–9; and previewing, 29, 64–65, 66; and undivided attention, 31. *See also* advocacy by parent; coaches; exclusion and expulsions; parents; school; teachers
advocacy, IEP/504, 147–49
advocacy, self-, 109–10, 192
advocacy by parent: and accommodations, 137–42, 146, 147–49, 156, 170–72; and bullying, 176–79, 185, 189–90, 192, 193–95; and child expression, 86–90; and exclusion, 51–56; and homeschooling, 159–60; and internalized ableism, 31; and protecting child from social policing, 80–84, 97, 98; and safety, 178–79; and school choice, 156–60; and treatments and therapies, 97, 98; and trust, 56, 156–60, 170–72, 189

217

neuroaffirming approaches: and previewing, 65–67; treatments and therapies, 109–11, 112–13

neurodivergence: defined, 1, 19; diversity of, 5; and exploitation, x, xi–xii; as "fake," 116, 120–23; terms overview, 19–20; writing about, ix–xvi

neurodivergence of author: and ADHD, 124–25; and autism, xvi, 1, 2–3, 16, 17, 40, 43, 77, 83, 87–88, 124; and bipolar disorder, xvi, 1, 2, 133–34; and child psychiatrist, 25, 26–28, 41, 51; and Christmas, 57–58, 78, 190; and diagnosis, 4, 87–88; exclusions and expulsions, 25–28, 41, 51, 52–53, 55–56; and executive function, 39–40; and gifted programs, 136–37, 141; and masking, 32–33, 77, 80; and medication, 4, 123–25, 133–34; and meltdowns, 3, 57–58, 63, 68, 76–78, 80, 83, 190; and perspective on parenting, ix–xiii, xvi–xvii, 1–4, 9–10; and piano, 52; and previewing, 66–67; and school, 5–9, 52–53; and shutdowns, 3, 8; and social skills, 87–89, 173–76; and talkativeness, 26, 32; and trauma, 2–4; and treatments, 88

neurotypical: as term, 19–20; and previewing, 29, 64–65; and stimming, 93

normate, as term, 20

norms. See social norms

Omeiza, Kala Allen, 18, 112
organizational strategies, 38, 39–40, 41
O'Toole, Jennifer Cook, 69–70, 191–93

parents: and boundaries, 4, 9, 79, 109, 133, 169; bullying, addressing, 176–79, 185, 189–90, 192, 193–95; bullying, dismissal of, 175, 176, 183, 184, 187–88, 191–92; bullying by,

190–95; effects on, of attacks/exclusions on kid, 26, 28, 53–56; and hypervigilance, 73–75, 95, 191–94; and isolation, 10; neurodivergence of author and perspective on parenting, xii–xiii, xvi–xvii, 1–4, 9–10; and pressure to conform, 4, 5, 31, 51; respect for fathers vs. mothers, 76; and safety, 178–79; and social policing, 69–75, 95, 97–98, 113, 191–94; touchstone questions for, 27, 54; treatment schism with neurodivergent adults, 105–9. See also advocacy by parent; mom of author

pediatric conduct disorder, 27–28
piano, 51, 52
police violence, 82, 112
politicians, 13–15
previewing, 29, 36, 44–45, 59, 64–67, 79
Price, Devon, 77, 92–93
privacy: medical, 44–45, 119, 126; online, ix, xiii–xv
property damage, 27, 28, 54
PTSD, 103, 183, 184
punishment: and bullying by adults, 189; corporal, 186–87; and race, 151–52; and school, 32, 141, 151–52; and social norms, 90–91, 92; and socioeconomic status, 151–52; vs. understanding behavior, 193–94

race: and accommodations, 150–52; and autism, 18, 72, 112–13, 150–52; and camps, 49–50, 152; and diagnosis, 18, 87, 151; and emotional expression, 72, 112; and homeschooling, 169; and meltdowns, 72; public vs. private schools, 152; and punishment, 151–52; and research, 18; and risk of violence, 82, 112; and social policing, 71–72, 80, 112–13; and testing, 7–8
Rehabilitation Act of 1973, 145. See also 504 plans

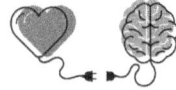

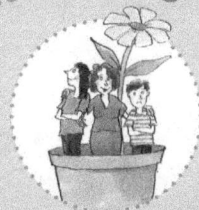